RETURN TO
BEAUTIFUL SKIN

*Your Guide to Truly Effective,
Nontoxic Skin Care*

Myra Michelle Eby
with Karolyn A. Gazella

Foreword by Mark Hyman, M.D.

**Basic
Health**
PUBLICATIONS, INC.

The information contained in this book is based upon the research and personal and professional experiences of the authors. It is not intended as a substitute for consulting with your physician or other healthcare provider. Any attempt to diagnose and treat an illness should be done under the direction of a healthcare professional.

The publisher does not advocate the use of any particular healthcare protocol but believes the information in this book should be available to the public. The publisher and authors are not responsible for any adverse effects or consequences resulting from the use of the suggestions, preparations, or procedures discussed in this book. Should the reader have any questions concerning the appropriateness of any procedures or preparation mentioned, the authors and the publisher strongly suggest consulting a professional healthcare advisor.

Basic Health Publications, Inc.
www.basichealthpub.com

Library of Congress Cataloging-in-Publication Data
Eby, Myra Michelle.
    Return to beautiful skin your guide to truly effective, nontoxic skin care /
Myra Michelle Eby with Karolyn A. Gazella.

    p. cm.
    Includes bibliographical references and index.
    ISBN 978-1-59120-229-5 (Paperback)
    ISBN 978-1-68162-777-9 (Hardcover)

    1. Skin—Care and hygiene. I. Gazella, Karolyn A. II. Title.

    RL87.E29   2008
    646.7'26—dc22

                                                          2007050841

Editor: Diana Drew
Typesetting/Book design: Gary A. Rosenberg
Cover design: Mike Stromberg

Contents

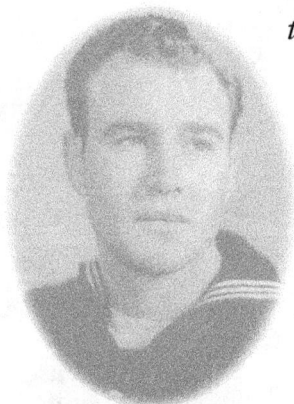

In loving memory of my father, John Adrian Mesko, the most humble, unselfish man I have ever known, and the one I had the privilege to call my Daddy.

Acknowledgments

I WOULD LIKE TO THANK MY FRIEND and coauthor, Karolyn Gazella, and my sister, Susan Mesko. Without their persistence, patience, and constant encouragement, this book would never have come to fruition. I also truly appreciate the support I have received from all of those connected with MyChelle Dermaceuticals, especially my sister Marian Hathorne.

I would like to thank my publisher, Norman Goldfind of Basic Health Publications, for having the confidence in my passion and vision to publish *Return to Beautiful Skin*. Many thanks, too, to my editor, Diana Drew, who was a delight and a pleasure to work with.

I certainly appreciate Dr. Mark Hyman's ringing endorsement of the concepts and approach to wellness that I take in this book.

And as the lights of my life, my husband, Chris, and our daughter, Winter Michelle, deserve unreserved thanks for their boundless love and support.

—Myra Michelle Eby

IT HAS BEEN AN HONOR WORKING with Myra Eby on this project. She is a true visionary and is most deserving of her unbridled success. I thank her for giving me this opportunity. Thanks also to our publisher, editor, and all of those involved with the creation of this book. Special appreciation, admiration, and love to Susan Mesko.

—Karolyn A. Gazella

Foreword

I have spent my professional medical career showing patients how to manage their health problems within an entirely new frame of reference. My goal is to help people understand and address the causes of illness, rather than just treating the symptoms.

To change medicine and fix a broken healthcare system, we must first feel empowered. *Return to Beautiful Skin* empowers readers by showing them how to make better choices when it comes to their body care products.

According to the coalition of nonprofit organizations known as the Environmental Working Group, every day one in five adults are exposed to cancer-causing ingredients in personal care products. On average, adults use nine different personal care products each day that have ingredients that can potentially contribute to illness.

As we enhance wellness through diet and lifestyle, we should also be evaluating all the products we use, including our skin care products. Our skin is the largest organ of the human body. Like a sponge, it can soak up toxins from the sun, the air, the food we eat, and, yes, even the products we use on it. Conversely, when the skin is in good condition it also protects us. Just like other key organs and systems in the body, our skin will be vibrant and healthy if we nourish and protect it.

In this book, the authors describe the importance of effectively nourishing and protecting your skin. There are helpful lists of ingredients to avoid, as well as information about nontoxic, therapeutic skin care ingredients. You will also learn how to customize your skin care routine. There are separate chapters on important issues, such as acne, sun care, and aging skin. Finally, the authors will teach you how to enhance the health of your skin from the inside out.

We are constantly bombarded with quick-fix antiwrinkle and skin care cures that don't work or only work temporarily. The authors of this book will show you how to *Return to Beautiful Skin* safely and permanently.

Myra and Karolyn have devoted their professional careers to the natural health industry. Myra is the president and founder of an innovative skin care company and is a leader in the field of dermaceutical development, safely combining the best of nature and science. Karolyn is the coauthor of the *Definitive Guide to Cancer*, as well as numerous articles and books. Together they create a powerful team to disseminate information about truly effective, nontoxic skin care.

If you want your skin to look and feel younger or you have a specific skin concern, this book is for you. I highly recommend it.

—Mark Hyman, M.D.
New York Times best-selling author of *UltraMetabolism*
and coauthor of *Ultraprevention*
www.drhyman.com

Introduction

L et's face it: We baby boomers have made it quite clear—we are committed to renewing and maintaining our skin's youthful glow. Just look at the millions of advertising dollars spent pushing skin care products, potions, and special surgeries. We are bombarded with messages on radio, on television, and in magazines. We are obsessed with our skin. Everything from acne to old age can cause a sane person to go mad, spending a fortune on products to smooth those worry lines, take away the shine, or soothe the dryness. It has been reported that we spend more on skin care products than we do on education. In a twenty-four-hour period, the average person uses about ten different cosmetic and personal care products, bolstering a multibillion dollar industry.

Skin care is everywhere. Numerous lotions line store shelves, celebrities push their signature products on the Home Shopping Network, and countless anti-wrinkle products proliferate online. It's confusing and can be overwhelming.

While it's hard to avoid the lure of quick fixes and miracle wrinkle cures, today's sophisticated consumer is tapping into her inner skeptic. I have talked to thousands of people over the years, and I've learned that most want more than false promises—they even want more than products that work. Certainly, they want the products they use to be effective, but they also want those products to be safe. I understand these demands because that's what I want, too! Although I'm the founder and president of my own skin care company, first and foremost, I'm a consumer, just like you.

I also know what it's like to be upset by what the morning mirror reflects. I know what it's like to be self-conscious and frustrated. Here is my story.

MYRA'S STORY

I understand firsthand how devastating it can be to have unhealthy skin. As a teenager, I developed mild acne, which continued to worsen with age until I reached my mid-thirties. Being the object of ridicule by other kids was horrible. As a young adult, I was ashamed of my acne breakouts. It was utterly unbearable. I spent many years being shy and feeling ugly.

Unfortunately, my story is the norm. Our skin is not only the largest organ of the body it is also the most visible. We humans tend to judge others by the first glimpse we have of them, and we judge ourselves by the reflection staring back at us in the mirror.

Every morning I hoped to see calmer, smoother skin on my face, only to find yet another acne lesion. I fasted, detoxed, and cleansed—with no improvement. I tried every acne product I could find, only to be disappointed time and time again. I became so frustrated that I decided to take control of the situation myself. I found that when I made my own skin care concoctions in the kitchen blender, with fresh fruits, yogurt, and honey, I always saw an immediate calming and soothing effect. This led me to develop more home recipes. The drawback was that I had to make these fresh every day, which was neither practical nor efficient. I was also missing one key element—concentrated bioactive ingredients.

While I worked in the holistic health industry all my adult life, I felt I was not the perfect "poster child" for holistic living because of my flawed skin. I was always searching for that special product that would help make my skin radiant. Finally, after twelve years of working as an educator and salesperson for several different holistic health companies, I decided to create my own skin care company. I knew I wanted to use only the highest-quality, active ingredients, in formulations based on cutting-edge science, and I vowed never to use potentially toxic ingredients. I loved the idea of kitchen cosmetics with a scientific twist—so I decided to go for it.

As a wife and mother, I can relate to the frustrations voiced by women who can't find truly natural skin care products that work for them and their loved ones. I have been frustrated, too! After spending years concocting my own natural skin poultices and masks, using my blender and ingredients I found in my refrigerator, I decided to channel my energy into something that could help others get the same benefits I was achieving. In 2000 I created MyChelle Dermaceuticals, an all-natural, eco-friendly, cruelty-free skin care company. It has been an entrepreneurial dream come true!

I have spent more than twenty-five years educating people about natural products. The use of irritating, toxic chemicals in skin care products has always troubled me, especially because most people aren't even aware of how dangerous some of the most common ingredients are. These toxic ingredients will not fulfill their promise of keeping you looking beautiful and radiant. Long term, they will also have devastating effects on your skin, your health, and our environment.

I am on a mission to expose the dark side of the personal care products industry. I have always believed that an educated consumer is a healthier consumer, and that applies to skin care consumers, too.

Skin is a significant part of who we are—not only physically, but emotionally as well. Our skin can have a negative or a positive impact on our moods and confidence levels. By using nontoxic, highly effective, natural skin care products, we can create a self-assured, healthy reflection in the mirror each day.

I have joined forces with my friend and accomplished health writer, Karolyn A. Gazella, to create this definitive guide to truly effective, nontoxic skin care. My goal is to give readers trustworthy, comprehensive information about skin care. You will learn what it means for a product to be natural, and how to create a nontoxic skin care regimen that's also very effective, drawing on the best natural, bioactive ingredients and cutting-edge science available today. I will provide you with lists of ingredients to avoid, as well as must-have ingredients. I'll help you customize your skin

care plan based on your special needs and your individual skin type. And, finally, I will teach you how to take care of your skin from the inside out.
As a skin care consumer, you should demand a program that is safe and effective. This book will teach you how to get both.

KAROLYN'S STORY

Two days after I turned thirty-three, I underwent surgery for ovarian cancer. In an instant, my life changed, and so did my skin. Overnight, I had become a menopausal woman. The doctor had flipped the switch, and my body struggled to figure out how to manage without estrogen. Chronologically, I was only thirty-three, but that's not what my body thought. Without ovaries, my body was not getting the estrogen it needed so it "assumed" that I was fifty-three, not thirty-three.

I experienced most of the common symptoms of menopause. That first year was the most difficult: insomnia, depression, loss of libido, vaginal dryness, night sweats, hot flashes, and dry—very dry—skin. Before my surgery, my skin always had that healthy Midwest glow—not too oily and never dry. After surgery, that glow was gone. As I managed all my symptoms, I had to figure out some way to recapture my youthful skin.

The menopausal experience can vary dramatically for women. Some women experience one hot flash and they're done. Others experience symptoms that substantially disrupt their lives. When menopause is surgically induced, as mine was, it can come with more challenging symptoms.

My story gets a little more complicated because I'm at very high risk of developing breast cancer as a result of my family history. In fact, our family has the breast-ovarian cancer gene. My sister was diagnosed with breast cancer and less than six months later, my mom died of advanced pancreatic cancer. My cancer came less than three months after my mom died. That's three cancers in eight months in one family! In addition, I have had several aunts and first cousins who have been diagnosed with breast cancer.

Because of my family history, hormone replacement therapy to manage my menopausal symptoms was out of the question. I use an all-natural approach to ease my menopausal symptoms. Fortunately, this natural approach has also helped me prevent a cancer recurrence. Through a combination of diet, exercise, nutritional supplements, and a mind-body-spirit approach to health, I am able to control my menopausal symptoms and boost my body's ability to heal and stay healthy. And guess what? My skin has reaped the benefits.

Early on in my search for ways to stay healthy, I learned that I needed to focus on all-natural, nontoxic skin care products. In this book, Myra explains the dangers of common toxic skin care ingredients. As a person concerned about cancer, I paid special attention to Myra's advice about avoiding estrogen mimickers and other toxins in common personal care products. She explained that these toxins mimic estrogen activity in the body and can be just as carcinogenic as excess estrogens in our food and the environment.

I am happy to report that in 2008, I celebrated my thirteenth year of being cancer free. At age forty-six, I feel more vibrant and healthy than ever.

In addition to our own stories, this book includes stories of some of the people Myra has talked to over the years. You'll read about their struggles and how they overcame their skin challenges. These are people just like me and you—people whose lives Myra has changed for the better.

I have known Myra Eby for more than fifteen years. I started in the natural health industry as the marketing director for a national supplement manufacturer. Back then, Myra was one of the company's leading salespeople. We became fast friends. We've stayed in touch over the years, I've watched her progress, and I've applauded her success.

I choose my writing projects carefully, and when Myra approached me about helping her with this book, I didn't hesitate. I wanted to work with a good friend but I also wanted to be associated with a project of high integrity, and that's what Myra has always represented to me. She is passionate about this topic and I knew that together we could create something that could potentially help many people. When we first talked about this book, I was excited about working on it because I felt it could make a difference for all those people confused about how to improve their skin. I'm proud of what we've created and we hope that as you fine-tune your skin care routine, you find this book to be a valuable guide.

MIRROR IMAGE

We often take our skin for granted until there's a problem—acne, wrinkles, dryness, or blemishes. But our skin is a significant part of who we are. What we see in the mirror often sets the tone for the day. The health of our skin can influence our mood and confidence levels. After decades of research, I have found that by using nontoxic, effective, natural skin care products, we can have vibrant, younger-looking skin. All of us can see the radiant image in the mirror—the one we've been searching for all these years.

But before we can identify the components of a safe and effective skin care plan, we need to understand the skin. What is skin? How does it regenerate and how can we rejuvenate it? And why is it so important to protect the health of our skin?

1 *Your Shell*

The skin is not just the body's wrapper. While it's true that the skin is the outermost layer between you and your environment, it is much more than just a simple cover for your bones and organs. The skin is the largest organ of the body. You may not think of the skin as an organ, but it is, and it plays an essential role in overall health.

Not only does our outer shell encase us, it serves many significant functions including:

🐾 Protecting us from injury and parasite invasion

🐾 Providing us with our sense of touch

🐾 Regulating our body temperature and preventing dehydration

🐾 Aiding in detoxification and elimination

🐾 Assisting with vitamin D synthesis when it's exposed to sunlight

🐾 Helping our immune system fight infection

Yes, the importance of our skin goes way beyond wrinkles and age spots. Our skin comprises an intricate array of cells and systems that work together to keep us vibrant and healthy while contributing to our overall wellness.

IT'S ALIVE

Our skin weighs approximately eleven pounds (5kg) and measures about twenty-one square feet ($2m^2$) as it wraps its way around our bodies. The skin's blood vessels, nerves, and various glands make this one of the most complex organs in the human body. The skin of the average adult contains around two hundred sweat glands and thirty sebaceous (oil) glands. The thickness of the skin varies, depending on its location in the body. The skin on the face—particularly under the eyes, eyelids, and on the lips—is the thinnest of all, and therefore the most vulnerable.

Our skin is alive and dynamic. It is always changing and regenerating itself, though at different rates, depending on our age. Infants regenerate skin cells in as few as fourteen days. By the time we reach middle age, it can take about thirty-five days to generate new skin cells. On average, the life cycle of a skin cell is twenty-eight days. In fact, the skin grows faster than any other organ in the body. At this moment, your skin is creating, growing, and regenerating millions of new skin cells.

There are two distinct layers of the skin: the epidermis, or the outer layer, and the dermis. The dermis, which is located just under what we refer to as the *skin*, contains the nerves that give us the ability to feel changes in our environment, including heat, cold, pain, and pressure, plus the sensation associated with touch. The dermis also connects blood vessels to the base of the epidermis. (*Note:* Skin care terms and definitions are featured in Appendix A at the back of the book.)

Most skin cell activity and metamorphosis takes place in the skin's outer layer, the epidermis. There are five layers within the epidermis. From the bottom up, those layers are:

1. stratum germativum (commonly called the basal layer)

2. stratum spinosum

3. stratum granulosum

4. stratum licidum

5. stratum corneum

Specialized skin cells work their way up from the bottom layer to the top basal layer.

Melanocytes are cells located in the base of the epidermis. These cells produce melanin, which is a dark pigment that helps create the color of our skin. Although we all have the same number of melanocyte cells, the amount of melanin our body produces is genetically controlled. Skin color is determined by melanocyte activity, which is influenced by our genes, the environment, and a number of physiological factors. Because sunlight stimulates the production of melanin, I'll discuss it in more detail in Chapter 7. Melanocytes are just one of the many types of cells located in our skin.

As mentioned previously, a skin cell's life cycle begins at the bottom of the epidermis, also known as the basal layer. This is where the cells receive nutrients via blood so they can actively divide and grow. The formation of new cells causes the older cells to be pushed up through the layers of the epidermis, eventually making their way to the skin's surface. As these older cells are pushed up, they receive less moisture and fewer nutrients so by the time they reach the top they are flat and dead. (For more information on the different layers and cells of the skin, see the illustration below.)

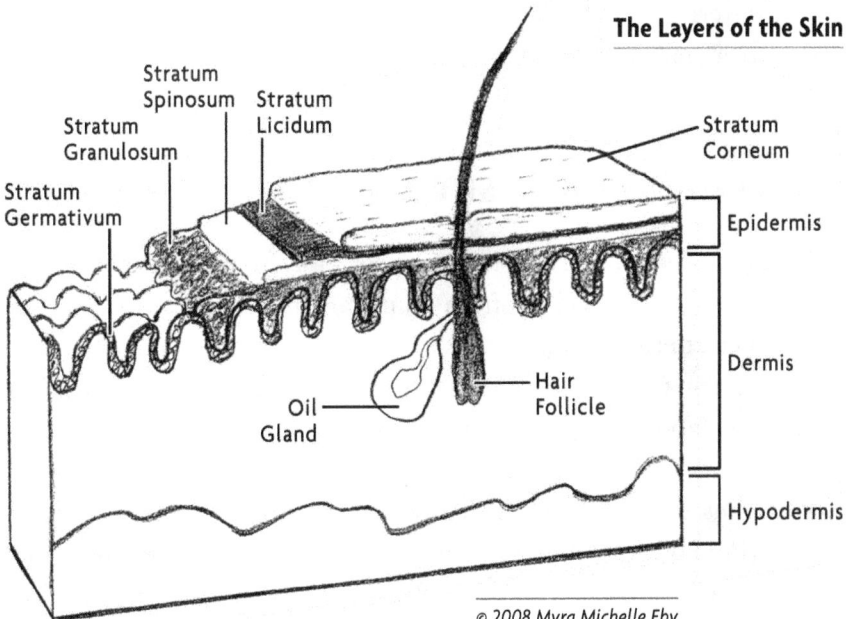

The Layers of the Skin

Stratum Spinosum
Stratum Licidum
Stratum Granulosum
Stratum Germativum
Stratum Corneum
Epidermis
Dermis
Hypodermis
Oil Gland
Hair Follicle

© 2008 Myra Michelle Eby

When skin cells are born, they are filled with fluid and very plump. I like to compare them to juicy grapes. These cells share space with collagen and elastin, the supportive fibers and protein that give skin its youthful elasticity. Many factors reduce our body's production of collagen and elastin, including genetics, age, the environment, and our lifestyle. (For more on lifestyle factors, see Chapter 9.) As collagen and elastin production declines, skin begins to sag. And because of the increasing lack of moisture as they are pushed up the epidermis, skin cells also become dehydrated. Reduced collagen production and dehydration are two key contributors to the accelerated aging of the skin.

Accumulated dead cells make up the top layer of the skin which is the outermost layer of the epidermis. Depending on its location in the body, this dead skin layer may be thin—only a few layers of cells deep, such as in the scalp—or thick, as many as fifty cells deep in places like the palms of the hands and the soles of feet. Eventually, the dead cells become detached as they slough off, making room for the cells below them. By the time you celebrate your fortieth birthday, this process has taken place more than five hundred times. In fact, it has been estimated that about 90 percent of household dust is made up of dead skin cells.

Bolstering the process of effective skin cell repair and rejuvenation will help create radiant skin. It will also contribute to the overall health of your skin so it can carry out all its important functions.

PROTECTION AND SUPPORT

One of the key roles of the skin is to protect us from our external environment. Our skin defends us from injury, environmental assault, parasites, and other external invaders.

The skin is one of the most sophisticated sponges ever created. That sets up a "good news–bad news" scenario. The bad news is that once a chemical has penetrated the outer layer of our skin, it can easily move into the dermis, where there is a rich blood supply ready to take it anywhere deep within the body. The good news is that the skin can also help detoxify these same toxic chemicals. The skin can transform toxins into benign substances that can be excreted through urination and through the skin when we sweat. The skin produces enzymes that can convert chemicals it's exposed to into water-soluble molecules so they can be eliminated more easily. These transformed toxins, now neutralized so they cannot harm us, can then be excreted through the skin when we sweat or in our urine. It is estimated that about 450 grams of toxins are excreted through our sweat each day. Regular use of saunas, steam baths, and hot baths, can promote this type of detoxification.

Exercise is a great way to produce sweat and discharge toxins, especially those stored in fat tissues. Aerobic exercise, in particular, promotes this process because it also increases the flow of oxygen throughout the body. Oxygenation helps the skin look and feel healthy. Using a loofah or skin brush after a sauna or an aerobic workout will help remove dead skin cells, unblock pores, and increase circulation in the skin. It's also very important to cleanse your face after a vigorous workout or after spending time in a sauna or a steam bath.

Our skin regulates body temperature and is instrumental in protecting us from dehydration. We humans are warm-blooded, which means we have the ability to maintain a consistent internal body temperature no matter what the external conditions. This is critical because proper enzyme and organ function requires an ideal internal temperature. Our internal body temperature cannot vary too much or we will suffer serious consequences. If our body temperature fluctuates dramatically, we may experience muscle failure, loss of consciousness, problems with our central nervous system, and even death. When we get overheated, we begin to perspire and that has a cooling effect. When we are cold, the tiny muscles around the hair follicles all over the skin stiffen up and and cause the shorter hairs to stand out,

DID YOU KNOW?

The reason your fingers and toes wrinkle when you are in the bathtub is because the outermost layer of the skin swells as it absorbs water and then compensates by wrinkling.

providing greater insulation from the external cold. This stiffening of the muscles is what we know as "goose bumps" and when this happens we can experience the sensation of shivering, which is another attempt by the skin to keep us warm. So, as you can see, this amazing organ possesses an inherent ability to help protect us from hyper- and hypothermia.

One often-overlooked aspect of our skin is its connection to immunity. In addition to the blood vessels, glands, and cells, there are also specialized immune-system cells scattered throughout the skin. Just as with other cells in the body's immune system, these special immune-system skin cells can detect bacterial or viral invaders and destroy and remove them before they do any harm.

According to German researcher Thomas Schwarz, Ph.D., "The skin does not only function as a mechanical barrier but also uses the immune system for protection." That is, the skin can help fight infection and help our wounds heal.

Our skin plays a critical role in synthesizing vitamin D as well. Vitamin D is very important in maintaining proper bone health and works collaboratively with other vitamins and minerals to stimulate immunity. Recent research has even demonstrated that vitamin D can help prevent and treat some cancers, including breast, colon, and prostate cancer. When the skin is exposed to ultraviolet rays in sunlight, it can convert a precursor skin molecule into vitamin D. Keep in mind that while vitamin D plays a vital role in our health, it only takes a little sunlight to create enough vitamin D for optimum health, so you should not use the need for vitamin D as an excuse to overindulge in sunbathing without proper protection. Chapter 7 focuses entirely on sun care.

Of course, one of the most fascinating things our skin does is give us the sense of touch. Whether you are playing in the mud with your child, feeling the warmth of a loved one lying next to you, or holding a soft puppy, our feeling of touch is amazing and priceless.

Our skin gives us many gifts. It offers us protection from a toxic world. It helps us detoxify and eliminate substances we don't need. It supports immunity and keeps our body temperature well balanced. Now it's time for us to give our skin the support and care it needs.

A Child's Skin and the Sun

As mentioned previously, the skin cells of infants and young children regenerate more quickly than those of adults. Just like the child itself, the skin cells are young and vulnerable. A child's skin is also not as thick as that of adults and has not yet developed protective mechanisms. With age comes the ability to protect ourselves from a toxic environment. Children lack that ability. This is especially true when it comes to the sun. Sun damage early in life compromises the health of our skin cells as we age. Now more than ever, we must protect our children from the sun. The sun's rays are becoming more intense as the ozone layer becomes depleted and stressed. To give children the best opportunity for lifelong healthy skin and, even more important, to help them avoid skin cancer, we need to protect them from the sun. For more information about safe and effective sun protection, see Chapter 7.

IT'S UP TO US

If our skin is to protect and support us, we need to protect and support it in turn. There are many things to consider when we're trying to create and maintain the health of our skin. When we think of our skin, we should think about the many cells, glands, tissues, and systems that are at work inside this outer layer of the body. Let's not make their job any more difficult. Let's complement and enhance their activity so they can perform their tasks more effectively. This means avoiding toxins whenever possible. So choose skin care products that are not only effective but are also safe over the long term.

To help our skin be the best it can be, we need to address the following questions:

🦎 How can we identify unsafe ingredients and what are the health ramifications of those ingredients?

🦎 What does it mean to be *natural* and *nontoxic*? Why is that important?

🐾 How can we apply cutting-edge technology and science to create effective, yet safe skin care products?

🐾 Which nontoxic ingredients really work?

🐾 How can we support our skin in other ways?

🐾 How can we manage and ease challenging skin care issues?

🐾 How can we make sure that our skin care program is the safest and most effective regimen for our individual needs?

The following chapters will address these and many other important skin care dilemmas.

Aging Skin

While added years can confer wisdom and joy, our skin sometimes pays the price. What happens when our skin ages?

Here are just a few key changes that our skin can undergo as it ages:

• Collagen production declines and the number of elastic fibers decreases, causing the skin to sag.

• Oil-gland activity decreases, causing dry, itchy skin.

• Reduced fat tissue and sweat-gland activity can cause intolerance to cold and increased susceptibility to heat, impairing the skin's ability to regulate body temperature.

• And, finally, there can be a reduction in protection from ultraviolet light, increasing the risk of sunburn and skin cancer.

Sound bleak? Well, it doesn't have to be. Although certain changes in the skin are an inevitable part of the aging process, there are things you can do to help your skin age gracefully and healthfully. In Chapter 8, I will describe what you can do to help prevent the signs of accelerated aging skin.

Even though our skin is complex, our skin care routine doesn't have to be. We can support our skin by using information gleaned from the scientific literature to create a practical and simple daily skin care regimen.

MY PHILOSOPHY

Honoring our skin directly translates into respect for ourselves, our health, and the environment. Effective, natural skin care is not about being transformed into a Barbie doll. It's about doing the best we can for our skin and our overall health. In our effort to achieve vibrant, healthy skin, we also become healthier individuals, gain enhanced self-confidence, and promote our true beauty—beauty that begins on the inside, radiating throughout our lives.

Is it time for you to honor the skin you're in?

Along the Journey

Overwhelmed in Texas

Early on in my career, I was giving a lecture at a store in Texas. This was before I started to exclusively focus on skin care. I was discussing diet, lifestyle factors, and nutritional supplements to support the immune system. After I finished with my presentation, I asked if anyone had any questions. A middle-aged woman raised her hand timidly and I called on her.

"Frankly, I'm overwhelmed," she admitted. She went on to explain, "There's just too much. Too much information. Too many products. And it's all very frustrating. I find myself so overwhelmed that I just don't do anything."

This woman was paralyzed by the sheer magnitude of information out there. And here I was adding to her load.

"That's totally understandable and my sense is that many people in this audience feel the same way," I began. "But there are ways to evaluate and simplify the messages you are receiving." I told her how to assess the quality of information coming her way. I told her that she doesn't have to do everything perfectly every moment of every day.

"Be gentle with yourself and start out slowly. Just do one thing at a time. Before you know it, you'll be doing more than you ever expected." I told her about the 80/20 rule. "Try to make healthy choices 80 percent of the time and indulge if you like the other 20 percent."

Over the years I kept thinking back to this overwhelmed woman from Texas, because I continued to hear the same concern expressed over and over again. When it comes to health, most people are overwhelmed. If we give in to that feeling, however, we risk becoming complacent and doing nothing at all.

Recently, I read about a large survey conducted by the American Association of Cancer Research and the National Cancer Institute. According to the survey results, 70 percent of respondents said that they had heard about so many ways to prevent cancer that they were overwhelmed. Those same overwhelmed individuals said they felt as if there were nothing they could do about it, so they did nothing at all. This creates a self-fulfilling prophecy. Yes, cancer is a daunting illness, but research tells us that nearly 40 percent of all cancers are caused by a poor diet. So, in reality, there *is* something we can do to prevent it. Actually, when it comes to cancer prevention, there are many things we can do.

The same is true for skin care. Today when I lecture, I work to empower people about the proactive steps they can take to maintain healthy skin. Because we are bombarded with so much information, the next chapter features tips from Karolyn on how to evaluate health information. Karolyn's sidebar was adapted from her recent book, *Definitive Guide to Cancer*, which she cowrote with Dr. Lise Alschuler. I was proud to contribute a sidebar to her book, and now I'm excited to feature her information in this book (see page 29).

In addition, Chapter 9 offers practical information you can use to evaluate and change your diet and lifestyle to enhance the health of your skin.

2 *The Problem*

*I*n a fairly short period, we've managed to saturate our world with toxic chemicals. According to a report by Laura Orlando in *Dollars & Sense* magazine, before World War I, half of the United States' industrialized products were made from renewable plant-, wood-, and animal-based materials. By 2002, a whopping 92 percent of the materials used to make our products were synthetic and not renewable. Not only are many of these human-made materials dangerous to our health, the process used to produce them creates additional toxins.

"Few people understood the dangers to life that these new chemicals presented," explains Orlando. "Sickness and death among chemical manufacturing workers was sometimes the first indication that the material they worked with was toxic." Orlando also reports, "Among the most lethal of these products were synthetic pesticides."

Worldwide, pesticide production continues to be big business. The United States accounts for more than 20 percent of pesticide production and more than 25 percent of herbicide production. In the United States alone, more than 1.2 billion pounds (500 million kg) of pesticides are used each year. And that figure doesn't include wood preservatives and other toxic chemicals. It also doesn't include other harmful substances like lead, solvents, xenoestrogens/estrogen mimmickers (foreign estrogens), polychlorinated biphenyls (PCBs), and the many chemical by-products that are so liberally introduced into our environment, our water, and our food supply on a daily basis. Estrogen mimickers are especially harmful because they can cause cancer. They disrupt normal estrogen metabolism by occupying reserved estrogen receptor cites on our cells. This can lead to an excess pooling of estrogen in the body. There is a direct link between excess estrogen and certain cancers including breast, ovarian, and prostate.

Reports indicate that we share our daily lives with well over 75,000 different synthetic chemicals. According to *Nurture Nature Nurture Health*, by Mitchell Gaynor, MD, in 2000, U.S. manufacturers reported dumping 7.1 billion pounds (3.2 billion kg) of 650 different chemicals into our air and water. "The manufacturing [of these chemicals] goes unabated and the disposal of the chemicals has risen to worrisome (and unchecked) levels," Dr. Gaynor asserts.

We share our daily lives with well over 75,000 different synthetic chemicals.

There continues to be an overabundance of additives, preservatives, stabilizers, fillers, and fake ingredients in the products we consume and use in our everyday lives. Numerous chemicals have been created to make things look, smell, and taste more appealing. I love the ice cream commercial with the kids trying to pronounce those long chemical names on the ingredient label. The scientific literature is packed with studies demonstrating the link between chemicals known as persistent organic pollutants (POPs) and a variety of illnesses. (By the way, the term *organic* used to describe these chemicals is not the same as the term *organic* used to describe health-promoting foods.) High blood levels of POPs have been linked to cancer, diabetes and insulin resistance, arthritis (specifically rheumatoid arthritis), and learning disabilities and attention deficit disorder in children.

The products we use on our bodies have also fallen prey to this alarming and harmful trend. The U.S. Environmental Protection Agency (EPA) has identified five thousand different chemicals used in cosmetics alone. What's worse, body care products are not regulated as strictly as food. And because our skin is so absorbent and vulnerable to external, foreign chemicals, this issue is even more critical. Chemicals in our body care products can negatively impact our most important physiological functions, including:

🦁 our immune system (reducing immunity)

🦁 digestion and elimination (interfering with detoxification)

🦁 our endocrine system (upsetting hormonal balance and function)

"EDCs [endocrine-disrupting chemicals], which include many POPs, DDT, dioxins, PCBs, and phthalates, show up in cosmetics, pesticides, upholstery, and skin care products," reports Dr. Gaynor. "All have been shown to cause harm to each of our body systems."

FEELING EXPOSED

As I discussed in the first chapter, the skin performs many important tasks. It is one of the most fascinating and vital organs of the human body. But if we're not careful, the skin can also make us more vulnerable to illness. Just as it soaks up the sun, it will also absorb up to 60 percent of whatever it comes in contact with. That's right—anything that touches our skin has a chance of being absorbed by it. Once past the outside layer, the substance can move freely throughout the body. That's why it's so important to watch what we put on our skin. Fortunately, the opposite is also true. We can feed our skin nontoxic ingredients that actually nourish it.

Because body care products and cosmetics are most commonly applied directly to the skin, several watchdog organizations are finally beginning to shine a spotlight on the toxicity of body and beauty care products. A coalition of nonprofit organizations, known as the Environmental Working Group (EWG), has done extensive research in this area. Information released by EWG in June 2004 indicates that the average adult uses nine personal care products each day, containing a total of 126 unique and potentially dangerous chemicals. EWG reports that more than 25 percent of all women use at least fifteen personal care products daily.

Shockingly, EWG found that "one of every 13 women and one of every 23 men are exposed to ingredients that are known or probable human carcinogens [cancer-causing agents] every day through their use of personal care products." The organization further reports that one in five adults are potentially exposed to the top cancer-causing impurities found in personal care products every day. That's right: Ingredients commonly used in many body care products have been shown to cause cancer—yet millions of people slather these chemicals on one of the largest, most complex, and vital organs of the human body.

But let's face it: Nurturing our skin is no easy task. "We know that looking good not only makes us more attractive to others but also makes us feel good about ourselves," writes Kim Erickson in her book *Drop-Dead Gorgeous*. "And although, for most of us, the majority of products appear safe in the short run, the results from long-term use could be deadly."

We cannot put an end to smog, totally guard against ultraviolet radiation, or stave off age-related changes in the skin. We can, however, enhance our health and the health of our skin by avoiding toxins in the products we use on our skin.

BUYER BEWARE

"So, we primp, we perm, we powder—all without blinking a mascara-swathed eye," says Erickson. And if we do pay attention, we feel as if we need a biochemistry degree just to read the labels of the products we're using. The Food and Drug Administration (FDA) is the federal agency charged with policing these products. Lack of funding and staff, however, combined with high-powered, well-funded political lobbying from the cosmetics industry, makes monitoring these products a low priority for the FDA. As a result, no one is strictly monitoring the toxicity of the ingredients in these products. Essentially, we are on our own.

According to Dr. Gaynor, "Fewer than half of the applications [for new chemical compounds] to the EPA include any toxicity data, and the government approves most of these applications, some 80 percent, in less than a month."

Years ago, it was believed that regulating skin care products was not necessary because the skin provided a solid barrier that actually prevented the absorption of unsafe substances. The dawn of the transdermal drug delivery system (nicotine skin patches and birth control patches) has dispelled that myth and actually proven just the opposite. Our skin is, in fact, very absorbent. This is an example of how regulatory practice has failed to keep pace with scientific technology.

Many ingredients in the body care products used every day have been shown to be toxic. They can cause long-term damage to our overall health and also damage the skin. It's ironic that the ingredients in the very products consumers use to protect and enhance their skin are actually harming the skin.

The first step in protecting your skin is identifying and understanding ingredients that should be avoided. Here is a list of the most dangerous and most commonly used harmful body care product ingredients.

Ethylenediaminetetraacetic Acid (EDTA)

EDTA is a preservative for food and a common ingredient used in the cosmetics industry. EDTA is made from a number of toxic chemicals, including sodium cyanide, ethylenediamine, and formaldehyde. At one time, formaldehyde use was banned in the United States because of its toxicity. Limited concentrations can now be used, but it is not monitored very closely and there is no requirement for companies to list formaldehyde content on labels. Many European countries have either banned the use of formaldehyde completely or strictly enforce label descriptions, only allowing it to be used in very low concentrations. EDTA has been linked to heavy metal toxicity and may cause a variety of health problems including infertility, cancer, birth defects, and developmental delays in children.

FD&C and D&C Colorings

On the label, chemical colorings are noted as FD&C or D&C, followed by a number. These chemical colorings can be toxic to the body, overloading the liver and potentially triggering some cancers. These colors are made from coal tar. In its pure state, coal tar is poisonous. According to *Drop-Dead Gorgeous*, although coal tar colors designated as FD&C and D&C

were grandfathered into the 1938 Federal Food, Drug, and Cosmetic Act (that is, because they were already in use, they could remain in use), the World Health Organization considers them to be "probable carcinogens," meaning that they most likely cause cancer. "Unless a color additive receives a lot of publicity, as was the case with Red No. 2, most consumers are unaware of the impact that long-term use of coal tar colors can have on their health," explains Erickson. Color additives that have been banned or not approved for use include green 1, red 1, red 3, blue 6, and violet 2. Products that commonly contain these dyes include nail polish, shampoos, moisturizers and lotions, body cleansers, and deodorant. It's best to avoid all FD&C or D&C colors whenever possible.

Nitrosamines

We often think of nitrosamines as by-products of the food industry, most typically found in cured meats. However, nitrosamines can be formed when mixing chemicals in our body care products as well. According to Richard A. Scanlan, PhD, of the Linus Pauling Institute, there is a direct link between nitrosamines and cancer. It has been reported that shampooing with a product that contains nitrosamines can lead to absorption of this substance into the body in an amount that exceeds what would be absorbed after eating nitrate-containing foods. Nitrates in foods become nitrosamine once metabolized by the liver. There are several chemicals commonly used in body care products that can create nitrosamines, including diethanolamine (DEA), triethanolamine (TEA), monoethanolamine (MEA), formaldehyde, and sodium lauryl sulfate. The term *nitrosamine* will not be listed on the label, but sodium lauryl sulfate, MEA, DEA, and TEA may be listed there.

Nonylphenol

A surfactant (SURFace ACTive AgeNT) is a wetting solution commonly used in detergents because of its oil-dispersing properties. Nonylphenol is a surfactant used in body care products like shampoos, hair colors, and shaving creams. In addition, nonylphenol has estrogenic activities and can contribute to the development of estrogen-dependent cancers, such as breast, uterine, ovarian, and prostate. Even if nonylphenol is not added to the product, it has been shown that some chemicals including polyvinyl chloride (PVC) found in nail enamels can lead to the creation of nonylphenol. Nonylphenols have become commonplace in the food supply, as well as our environment. Although they cannot be avoided completely, they should be avoided in our body care products whenever possible.

Parabens

The scientific term for *parabens* is alkyl hydroxy benzoate preservatives. A wide range of these ingredients can be found in body care products in the form of ethyl-, butyl-, propyl-, and methylparaben. Adding one or more of these antimicorbial preservatives is an inexpensive way to increase shelf life. Chapter 4 features information about nontoxic, natural alternatives to parabens. Many scientific studies have confirmed that parabens have the potential to cause cancer because of their estrogenic activity. As mentioned previously, foreign estrogens in our environment, food, and many products (including skin care compounds) have been directly linked to the development of certain cancers, including breast, prostate, ovarian, and uterine. Because the liver needs to work even harder to detoxify these excess estrogens, these chemicals may contribute to other illnesses as well. The numerous adverse effects of parabens continue to be studied. Parabens can be found in a wide variety of body care products, including creams, lotions, and shampoos.

Petrolatum

Also known as petroleum jelly (brand name: *Vaseline*), as the name implies this clear, tasteless, odorless substance is derived from petroleum. According to the Environmental Working Group, petroleum jelly has been shown to contain a common contaminant known as polycyclic aromatic hydrocarbons (PAH). Animal studies have shown that PAHs can contribute to the development of breast tumors. It has been estimated that one out of every fourteen personal care products, including 15 percent of all lipsticks and 40 percent of all baby lotions and oils contain petrolatum.

Phenylenediamine

Phenylenediamine is a toxic compound found in some hair dyes. On the label it may be preceded by the letters m-, o-, or p-. Phenylenediamine has been shown to cause skin irritations, eczema, asthma, gastritis, and other health problems. This ingredient has also been grandfathered in and is protected under an FDA exemption adopted in 1938. There have been many attempts to remove this chemical from the market, or at least require strict package warnings; however, none of those attempts have been successful against the powerful cosmetics industry lobby. Phenylenediamine used in hair dyes has been successfully banned in Europe.

Phthalates

Pronounced THAY-lates, these chemicals are found in many personal care products. A dangerous aspect of phthalates is that they soak into the skin and accumulate over time. Just like parabens, phthalates disrupt estrogen metabolism, which can contribute to certain cancers. These chemicals are commonly found in hair sprays, perfumes, fragrances, and nail polish. Virtually all synthetic fragrances contain phthalates. These chemicals have been shown to build up in body fat. Phthalates have been linked to liver toxicity and genital malformation, and are thought to trigger some cancers. According to a study conducted by the Centers for Disease Control and Prevention in 2000, more than 75 percent of Americans tested had traces of phthalates in their urine. "Because the effects of these and other synthetic chemicals develop over the course of several decades, it's difficult to find a direct cause-and-effect scenario for certain chemical ingredients," Erickson points out. "A sixty-year-old woman who develops breast cancer wouldn't even think of blaming the makeup she's used every day for the past forty years." The most commonly used phthalates are di-2-ethyl hexyl phthalate (DEHP), diisodecyl phthalate (DIDP), and diisononyl phthalate (DINP).

Propylene Glycol

Propylene glycol and ethylene glycol are commonly used in antifreeze and de-icing solutions. They are also found in polyester, as well as paint and plastic solvents. Exposure to ethylene glycol is extremely dangerous. While propylene glycol is approved as a food additive and is used in the cosmetics industry, it is suspected of compromising the immune and respiratory systems, interfering with brain function, and (ironically) harming the skin. In the body care industry, propylene glycol is a cheap, moisture-carrying ingredient. Even though this ingredient is toxic, because of its low cost, it is often used in place of glycerin in many cosmetic and body care products. Interestingly, if you were to visit a manufacturing plant, you would see the required warning label stating AVOID SKIN CONTACT on the outside of the drums that contain propylene glycol. And yet, it is one of the most commonly used moisture-carrying ingredients in skin care products.

Sodium Lauryl Sulfate

A large number of body care products contain sodium lauryl sulfate, also called sodium laureth sulfate. Everything from lotions to toothpastes can contain this ingredient because of its lathering properties. About 90 percent of all products that foam contain this ingredient. Unfortunately, sodium lauryl sulfate is also a proven skin irritant. This ingredient can also lead to the formation of dioxin, a toxic compound. According to the FDA, dioxin can cause severe acne-like lesions that occur on the face and upper body. The FDA also reports that dioxin can cause skin rashes, skin discoloration, excessive body hair, mild liver damage, and, most disturbingly, it may cause cancer.

Synthetic Fragrances

Also known as synthetic musks, these chemical compounds have been shown to compromise cellular defense mechanisms that normally prevent toxins from entering the cells. National Geographic News and environmental organizations have reported that these fragrances are harmful to marine and animal life and most likely harmful to humans as well. Similar to phthalates, which are a common ingredient in synthetic fragrances, these chemicals accumulate in fat and can be dangerous. It has been estimated that a synthetic fragrance can contain as many as one hundred different chemicals. Toluene is commonly used in synthetic fragrances. Synthetic fragrances may include benzene derivatives and aldehydes, which both have been shown to cause severe allergic reactions, cancer, birth defects, and central nervous system disorders.

Talc

When you use talcum (talc) powders and sprays, it may seem as if you were doing something healing and refreshing for your skin; however, talc is highly toxic. According to the Fred Hutchinson Cancer Research Center, women who used talc regularly on their genital area had a much higher chance of developing ovarian cancer. Chemically, talc is similar to asbestos. In fact, it has even been shown to be harmful to the lungs when airborne. This makes talc body sprays just as dangerous as powders. According to the website preventcancer.com, "Cosmetic grade talcum powder is a carcinogen." My coauthor Karolyn developed ovarian cancer when she was just thirty-three years old. She told me that she used talc for years prior to her diagnosis. She didn't know about the dangers of this ingredient. While the talc she dusted on her body probably didn't directly cause Karolyn's cancer, we now know that it can be a contributing factor.

Urea

Urine from humans and animals creates urea. One of the most common uses of urea is as an ingredient in fertilizer. Urea is a preservative that has been shown to release trace amounts of formaldehyde into the skin, creating a toxic effect at the cellular level. Similar to polyester, this ingredient is known as a formaldehyde donor. As stated previously, formaldehyde is toxic; it can cause a variety of health problems, including joint pain. Imidazolidinyl urea and diazolidinyl urea, the most commonly used preservatives after parabens, are a primary cause of contact dermatitis. In addition to bovine urine, urea for body care products comes from wood alcohol. Neither is something I would want to put on my skin!

This list just barely skims the surface of the many chemicals to watch out for. My goal here is to spotlight the most dangerous of the body care chemicals that are in the products you may be using. Of course, it is absolutely critical to read the label of any product you buy very carefully.

BEYOND THE LABEL

Thanks to my mom, ever since I can remember I have always been a label reader. When I found out I was pregnant, I became an obsessive label reader. I wanted to be especially careful about my baby's exposure to toxic chemicals, preservatives, additives, and colorings. I was not only a meticulous label reader regarding the foods I ate, but also all products I used for my care. It was not easy in the beginning, but I soon developed a rhythm to my shopping and a high level of confidence in my ability to read labels. In addition, I came to trust certain manufacturers and avoided others. Label reading has become second nature to me, and it's a habit that I will now pass on to my daughter as she grows up. But the legacy of the label reader is just part of the picture. Reading the label is the easy part. It can be difficult to evaluate a product, however, if ingredients are omitted from the label. How can you make a decision if something is not even listed or if it's listed in unfamiliar terms?

Unfortunately, in today's "bottom line" society, some manufacturers deliberately fail to list all product ingredients on the label. They know that some consumers might not buy their products if they saw a long list of chemical additives on the label. Body care products are not regulated as strictly as foods, so many products actually contain toxic chemicals that are not listed on the label. While this provides a huge challenge for consumers, there are things you can do even if the label doesn't tell the whole story. Here are my suggestions on how to evaluate a product beyond the label:

🦋 **Your nose knows.** Trust your senses to help you determine if something is nontoxic. I like products that smell and look fresh, as if I could have them as a tasty snack before putting them on my skin. Products that have heavy perfume smells and unnatural-looking colors probably contain artificial ingredients and toxic fragrances.

🦋 **Divide and conquer.** If you are having a reaction to your skin care products even though the label specifies "all-natural," you should isolate the products and only use one at a time. You will then be able to determine which product(s) is causing the problem.

🦋 **Don't mix and match.** For consistent results, stick with products from the same manufacturer and choose a brand that you trust. It's also important to follow directions carefully and call the company's customer support line so you can get your questions answered.

🦋 **Build a relationship.** Get to know the product manufacturer. Be skeptical of companies that don't provide a toll-free number for consumers to call. It's important to have confidence in the manufacturer of the products you use.

🦋 **Cookie cutters are for cookies.** Remember, you are an individual with special skin care needs. A one-size-fits-all approach to skin care is not sustainable. I'll discuss more about individualizing your skin care plan in Chapter 5.

🦋 **Patience, please.** Do your research. Your skin care plan may not be perfect right away. Developing the safest, most effective skin care routine takes time and commitment. Have patience. Radiant skin will be your reward.

Reading the label is the first critical step to choosing the right skin care products. But that's just the beginning. Let your intuition and your results guide you beyond the label. It can also be difficult to evaluate health information on the web. The following section, "Evaluating Information Online," has been adapted with permission from the book *Definitive Guide to Cancer: An Integrative Approach to Prevention, Treatment and Healing*, by Lise Alschuler, ND, and Karolyn A. Gazella (Celestial Arts, 2007).

EVALUATING INFORMATION ONLINE

Many of us love to curl up with a juicy novel now and then. But when it comes to health information, fiction is the last thing we should be reading. Unfortunately, some online health information is fiction cleverly disguised as fact.

Here are some tips for evaluating health information on the web:

🐾 If the information is presented as educational or scientific, it should not be directly connected to product sales.

DID YOU KNOW?

Chemicals accumulate in the environment and in the body. Consider polychlorinated biphenyls (PCBs), which have been used in a wide variety of manufacturing plants, including those producing rubber and plastics. According to the EPA, even though PCBs were banned in 1977, approximately 70 percent of the chemicals that were made before that time are still in our environment more than thirty years later. PCBs have been found in humans and in our food supply. The EPA reports that clinical studies have linked PCBs to numerous health concerns, including cancer, neurological disorders, reduced sperm count, low birth weight in newborns, high blood pressure, and elevated cholesterol levels.

Toxic chemicals not only find a way to get into our bodies, they stay in. When absorbed through the skin, it can take years (even decades in some cases) for these chemicals to break down and be eliminated. The same is true for parabens, phthalates, and other chemicals found in many skin care products.

The EPA's "Dirty Dozen"

According to *Nurture Nature Nurture Health,* by Mitchell Gaynor, MD, the United States produces more than $300 billion worth of chemicals each year. "Currently, U.S. companies hold licenses to manufacture 75,000 or more chemicals for commercial use, and each year our government registers another 2,000 new chemicals," reports Dr. Gaynor.

In 2001, under pressure from the United Nations and other countries, the United States agreed to reduce and/or eliminate the production, use, and/or release of twelve persistent organic pollutants (POPs). This group of chemicals was informally known as the "dirty dozen." According to the U.S. Environmental Protection Agency (EPA), the "dirty dozen" can be found in these chemical categories:

- Insecticides, such as DDT, commonly used to control pests in agriculture and building materials.

- PCBs, used in hundreds of different commercial applications, including the manufacture of electrical products, paints, plastics, and rubber products.

- Chemical by-products, like dioxin, produced by waste incinerators and other industrial processes.

This effort does not even begin to scratch the surface when it comes to controlling the chemicals that are presently encroaching on our daily lives. According to the EPA, there are more than 3,200 chemicals added to foods, more than 1,000 chemicals added to consumer products, and over 5,000 chemicals in cosmetics alone. Cigarette smoke releases into the air 4,000 different chemicals. Perhaps this list needs to be expanded from the "dirty dozen" to the "grimy grand." Going from 12 to 1,000 chemicals as the target of a government crackdown would at least be a step in the right direction.

Body Care's "Dirty Dozen"

I've created my own "dirty dozen" of body care toxic ingredients. Gather together the lotions, soaps, shampoos, deodorants, sunscreens, and other body care products you use on a frequent basis. Are these ingredients listed on the product labels?

1. Ethylenediaminetretraacetic acid (EDTA)

2. FD&C and D&C synthetic colorings

3. Nitrosamines produced by DEA, TEA, MEA, or sodium lauryl/laureth sulfate

4. Nonylphenols produced by polyvinyl chloride

5. Parabens

6. Phenylenediamine

7. Phthalates

8. Propylene glycol

9. Sodium lauryl sulfate

10. Synthetic fragrances

11. Talc

12. Urea

These ingredients should be on your shopping "hit list." Although we may not be able to hunt down the purveyors of these nasty ingredients, we can certainly boycott them. It may take a little extra time, but it's possible to find body care products that do not contain these ingredients. Try to remove the "dirty dozen" from your shelves and replace them with nontoxic alternatives.

Check Out This Label!

Following are the ingredients listed on the label of a couple of common body care products. This first label is from a very popular moisturizing body lotion sold in most mainstream pharmacies and grocery stores. The front label of this product claims that it gives you "incredibly soft skin with jojoba oil and vitamin E." Let's take a look inside (this is the exact ingredient listing featured on the back of the label):

Water, myristyl alcohol, glycerin, mineral oil, butylene glycol, alcohol denat., stearic acid, petrolatum, myristyl myristate, glyceryl stearate, hydrogenated coco-glycerides, dimethicone, simmondsia chinensis (jojoba) seed oil, tocopheryl acetate, polyglyceryl-2 caprate, phenoxyethanol, lanolin alcohol, fragrance, carbomer, sodium hydroxide, methylparaben, ethylparaben, propylparaben, butylparaben, isobutylparaben.

- Notice that alcohol is the second ingredient and there are two other alcohols listed.

- Notice that this product contains five different types of parabens.

- This product also uses synthetic vitamin E (tocopheryl acetate), which is not nearly as effective as natural vitamin E (dl-tocopherol).

🐾 Articles and medical information should feature a credible author and author biography, or otherwise identify the source of the information. The author should disclose financial ties to product sales.

🐾 Scientific information, including research, clinical trials, case studies, protocols, and medical opinions, should be supported by a list of references.

🐾 Be wary of outlandish claims and theories associated with disease treatments.

🦎 Be sure the site and the information presented on the site are current.

🦎 Do not base your decision regarding credibility solely on patient testimonials.

🦎 Evaluate links just as critically as you evaluate the original site.

And How about This One?

The following label graces one of the best-selling body care products on the market today. It is a foaming face wash that claims it deep cleans, doesn't overdry, and is oil-free:

> Water, glycerin, sodium myristol sarcosinate, PEG-120 methyl glucose dioleate, sodium lauroamphaoacetate, aloe barbadensis leaf juice, polyquaternium-10, PEG-150 pentaerythrityl tetrastearate, glycol distearate, sodium laureth sulfate, cocamide MEA, laureth-10, disodium lauroamphodiacetate, sodium trideceth sulfate, citric acid, disodium EDTA, phenoxyethanol, DMDM hydantoin.

• This product contains two of the "dirty dozen" including MEA and EDTA.

• PEG is a plasticizing agent that has been shown to cause cancer in laboratory animals.

• Polyquaternium-10 releases formaldehyde.

• DMDM is a preservative that contains formaldehyde.

Just reading these ingredient lists is a real eye-opener. It certainly does not take a biochemist to recognize the "unnatural" and toxic chemistry of the ingredients listed on these labels. Put these labels (and the many others out there) next to a nontoxic label to compare. The difference will be dramatic.

🐾 Find out who runs the site and who pays for it. If the site is operated and paid for by a product manufacturer, the information may be biased.

🐾 You should be able to easily contact the site manager, owner, or key representative when you need clarification on issues associated with the site.

There is a great deal of quality information on the web that is not tied directly to products. One reliable source is PubMed, an online library of peer-reviewed and scientifically credible medical journals sponsored by the Library of Congress. Many universities and integrative health clinics also have quality information on their sites.

Some skepticism of both conventional and alternative health information online can be healthy. The web should not be your only resource when making health decisions. It's important to get other opinions regarding the data you glean from the web. The Internet has proven to be a valuable tool and a great technological advance. Caution should be exercised, however, when evaluating the millions of health websites presently online.

THE SOLUTION

Yes, our world is being inundated with chemicals. But there is no need to continually soak our skin in toxins. Lack of regulation of body care products may make our job a little more difficult, but we do have choices. The key is to become a meticulous label reader, while trusting your gut instinct. If a product contains one of the known toxins listed in this chapter, avoid that product. If a product contains an ingredient you are unfamiliar with or concerned about, do a little research. If you can't confirm beyond a shadow of a doubt that the ingredient is, in fact, nontoxic, avoid it.

It can be challenging to have perfect skin in an imperfect world, but it is possible. By focusing on natural, nontoxic ingredients, we will ensure that our skin and our overall health is the best it can be. But what exactly does it mean to be natural? We'll explore that concept in more detail in the next chapter.

Along the Journey

At Wit's End in Wisconsin

I have talked to a lot of frustrated people over the years. They are frustrated because they are doing everything they can and still not finding the answers they need—still not achieving the healthy, vibrant skin they long for. I vividly remember a conversation with a woman from Wisconsin who was near tears as she told me her story. She was a high school teacher in her mid-thirties. She said she always had beautiful skin and never had any problems until she turned thirty. She said nothing had changed in her routine and she had been using the same products for more than a decade. "My skin literally changed overnight," she said. One morning she woke up with dry, wrinkled skin around her eyes and even more dry, flaking skin around her mouth. For the past several years, she had the same intermittent and ongoing problems with the skin on her face.

I told her that I thought she was allergic to one or more of the synthetic ingredients in the products she was using. "But how can that be?" she asked in a frustrated tone. "I've been using these products almost my entire adult life."

I explained to her that it takes years, sometimes decades, for these ingredients to build up in a person's system to the point where they cause symptoms and/or physical damage. I also told her that as we age, our skin becomes more vulnerable and can no longer protect us from the toxic effects of these chemicals. In addition, they weaken our immune system, which causes us to become more sensitive to these universally used chemicals. "But I am really careful about the products I use on my face in particular," she said. Some products, I explained, may contain toxic ingredients but they may not be listed on the label.

"If that's the case, how do I know what's causing the problem?" she asked.

"You have to start all over again," I advised. I told her to discontinue using all her products. She needed to create an entirely new skin care routine and she needed to start with the basics. I gave her some of my recipes for home-made poultices, masks, and facial treatments. I also told her to introduce only

DID YOU KNOW?

In the United States, there are no regulations that force manufacturers of extracts to fully disclose to the final manufacturer of skin care formulations the use of potentially toxic, transient ingredients such as parabens, phthalates, EDTA, and the like. Look for ingredients listings with fully disclosed INCI (International Nomenclature of Cosmetic Ingredients) classifications in accordance with the Personal Care Products Council and EU-approved.

nontoxic products back into her routine very slowly, using one product at a time for at least five days. It seemed like a slow process but she was willing to do anything.

I received a letter from her about six months later: "Thank you so much! Finally, I am no longer frustrated with my skin. My skin looks better today than it did when I was in my twenties."

If skin care products were regulated as closely as foods, consumers might have an easier time determining which products to use and which to avoid. Unfortunately, that's not the case. This means that people who develop reactions to their skin care products may need to be patient and start from scratch. Through a process of elimination, you will be able to find effective, nontoxic products that work for you.

3

The Meaning of "Natural"

or more than two decades I have been involved in the natural health industry. Even before I started working in the industry, I was committed to maintaining a natural and holistic lifestyle. Thanks to my mom, when I was just twelve years old, I started eating a healthy diet. Because of her influence, I was a granola-eating, organic-food shopping, supplement-taking hippie at a very young age. I do spring cleanses, I drink wheat grass, and I buy organic whenever it's available. Over the years, I have supported the natural foods industry while trying to get even more people to embrace natural approaches. So eating natural foods and adopting disease prevention strategies are huge parts of my life.

Yet, I have been asking myself recently, what does it really mean to be *natural*? The word has become a cliché—almost devoid of meaning. It's sad when I think of the power and influence the word used to have. To me, *natural* is synonymous with *nontoxic*. Today, however, it's vastly overused and has been hijacked by manufacturers who don't even know what it means to live a natural life. Remember one of the product labels in the last chapter? That well-known brand manufacturer decided to jump on the "natural" bandwagon by adding minuscule amounts of jojoba oil and vitamin E to its moisturizer. And yet, the product still contains numerous ingredients that are toxic. Product ingredients are listed in the order of greatest to least amounts used in manufacturing the product, with the most prominent ingredients at the beginning of the list. The jojoba oil and vitamin E are listed far below the chemicals. The reality is, upon close inspection, that product isn't natural at all. Don't feel bad: I myself was a victim of these so-called "natural" products, thinking I was using safe, effective skin care preparations. No more!

Here are a few more examples of products claiming to be natural, while they're nothing of the sort:

🙊 A popular brand of shampoo with *herbal* in its name incorporates chamomile, aloe vera, and passion flower in its shampoos, yet they also contain EDTA, DMDM, and three different FD&C and D&C coal tar colors.

🙊 A mainstream chain's brand of shower gel adds orange blossom and cotton extracts but also contains DEA as a third and TEA as a fourth ingredient; this product also contains four different coal tar colors, EDTA, and parabens.

🙊 The manufacturer of a popular moisturizer proudly proclaims on the front label, NOW WITH SHEA BUTTER, but the product still contains the same other toxic ingredients that it always had, including parabens and added synthetic fragrances and coal tar colorings.

So, what actually constitutes a product that's *natural*? More important, how can consumers who want natural products tell if they are getting a truly natural product?

NATURAL AND NONTOXIC

Webster's dictionary defines *natural* as being "present in or produced by nature," as opposed to being produced synthetically. But natural is not just simply adding an ingredient or two from nature. Natural is much more than that. The word *natural* should indicate that all ingredients are derived from nature, rather than solely from synthetic processes. (Keep in mind that not all synthetic processes are toxic: Synthesized ingredients may still be considered natural. Many natural vitamins, for instance, are grown in the lab.) *Natural* means using ingredients from nature that are not only appropriate for the application but also included at the right dosage and molecular structure. Unfortunately, being natural is not regulated in this context. There are no rules that apply to using this term in marketing and on labels for cosmetics or body care products.

To help people understand what *natural* is, I now always pair that word with *nontoxic*. Natural is nontoxic, and nontoxic is what we need and what natural represents to most people. And if I had to choose one word over the other, I'd choose *nontoxic*. We are looking for products that are not toxic—safe for us to use, safe for our families, and safe for our environment.

OK—back to Webster's. *Toxic* means "harmful, destructive, or deadly." There can be toxic actions, toxic relationships, toxic people, and toxic products. The ingredients discussed in the previous chapter certainly fall into the category of toxic. Therefore, a product that is nontoxic does not contain toxic ingredients. A toxin is a poisonous substance that can harm living tissues. The many toxic ingredients being added to body care products unequivocally fall into the category of potentially harmful substances.

We've established that *nontoxic* means *natural* and *natural* means *nontoxic*, but how can we determine if a product is nontoxic? Look beyond the one or two ingredients spotlighted on the front of the label. Never rely on just the front label to give you the information you need. Turn products around and look at the ingredients listed on the back. Even if there is a long, unrecognizable ingredient that is natural, the manufacturer should put the common name (typically an herb) in parenthesis. Here's an example of how that will look:

> *Butyrospermum parkii* (shea butter)
>
> *Papaver rhoeas* (red poppy)
>
> *Punica granatum* (pomegranate)
>
> *Citrus paradisa* (pink grapefruit)
>
> *Zingiber officinale* (ginger)
>
> *Rosa rubiginosa* (rose hips)

Even if the Latin herbal name is used, as these previous examples illustrate, the common name should be in parenthesis so the consumer knows what that ingredient is. For more information on body care ingredients, see Appendix B, "Nourishing Ingredients," at the back of this book.

There is no question that reading labels can be tricky and it would take years of training to recognize and understand the action of all of the more than five thousand different chemicals used by the body care and cosmetics industry. However, it may be helpful to follow these two rules:

1. If the ingredient listed on the product is featured in the previous chapter (or an ingredient that is similar to those listed in the *Dirty Dozen* lists featured on pages 30 and 31), you should avoid that product.

2. If the majority of the ingredients are from natural sources that are easily identified, you may want to consider using that product.

It's always wise to do your homework before you decide on skin care products. If you see any ingredients on the label that are hard to pronounce, or are expressed in unfamiliar terms, get in touch with the company and determine for yourself if that product is nontoxic. As a conscious and conscientious consumer, it is your responsibility to investigate and feel comfortable with the products you're using.

ORGANIC INGREDIENTS

In the early 1970s, the natural foods industry pioneered the concept of organic foods. Decades ago, organic products were just one part of a grass-roots natural health movement. Buying organic, however, is no longer a cottage industry reserved for hard-core health enthusiasts. Purchasing organic products has become much more common and is an increasingly popular trend. Today, we can even get organic ingredients in our body care products.

According to the Organic Trade Association (OTA), "*Organic* refers to the way agricultural products are grown and processed." Organic farmers and ingredient producers make sure they replenish the soil, rather than deplete it, while avoiding the use of toxic pesticides and fertilizers. In the case of milk and meat products, organic farmers also do not use growth hormones and they feed their animals organic feed.

"Organically produced foods also must be produced without the use of antibiotics, synthetic hormones, genetic engineering and other excluded practices, sewage sludge, or irradiation," explains the OTA. "Organic foods are minimally processed without artificial ingredients, preservatives, or irradiation to maintain the integrity of the food."

The surge in sales of organic foods demonstrates the strong consumer demand for this healthy alternative. In fact, *Organic Monitor* magazine reports that worldwide sales of organic food and drinks reached $23 billion in 2002. Sales of organic products in North America have finally surpassed total sales of organics in Europe. Statistics from the USDA for 2003 showed that 73 percent of conventional grocery stores carried organic products and that these products were also available in nearly twenty thousand natural food stores.

Fortunately, some manufacturers of skin care products are recognizing the benefits of adding organic ingredients to their products as well. Primarily, this trend in body care involves the use of organically grown herbs and whole-food concentrates. Organically grown herbal extracts not only provide the benefit of the herb but also the assurance that the herb was produced in a more health-promoting manner that's also better for our environment. I advocate, promote, and use organic products whenever possible.

The system used to monitor adherence to organic regulations is not perfect, but we've come a long way over the years. As these products and ingredients become more popular, I certainly hope the government will do a better job of policing this industry.

"Beyond the direct benefits to consumers eating organic foods, organic farming practices are easier on the earth," noted food scientist and natural health consultant Mary Mulry, PhD. "Conventional agriculture can contaminate more than the food that is grown; it can contribute to pollution of the air, soil, and water."

ENVIRONMENTALLY SAFE

When we think of environmental toxins, we think of the more than 75,000 different chemicals produced in North America each year, some of which were mentioned in Chapter 2: pesticides, solvents, preservatives, dioxin, and others. We don't often think of toxins in our body care products. At least I didn't, until one day while I was camping, and I had an "ah-ha" moment.

I am a very active person. I like to ski, bicycle, hike, and camp. I remember one camping trip in particular. It was years ago, before I had started my own skin care company. We chose a picturesque remote area in northern Arizona, on the Mogollon Rim. We hiked into a private campsite that was next to a clear-running stream. It was August and still hot enough to appreciate that cool running water. I woke up early the first morning of our trip and went to the stream to wash my face. As I lifted my cleanser out of my bag, I thought about those surroundings: that wonderful stream running happily across a beautiful vista. In that moment, I wondered if it was safe to wash my face—not because the stream was unsafe, but because I was worried about whether the product I was using was safe for the stream, the ecosystem, the fish, the animals that drank out of the stream, and the environment overall.

Yes, I washed my face in the stream but as soon as I got back from that trip, I researched the environmental issues associated with the ingredients in the skin care products I was using. After all, I thought, if it's unhealthy for the stream, it's probably unhealthy for me.

Body care is not only what goes on the body but also what goes down the drain. How many toxins are created in producing these universally used chemicals? I'm concerned about our environment and I don't want to add to the burden. The products I use need to smell and look fresh; they need to come from natural, nontoxic sources. They also need to be harvested or extracted in a manner that is respectful of our environment. And I'm not alone in my view. Increasingly, consumers are looking at the big picture when making their product choices. This sense of consciousness will make the world a better place for my daughter and the generations to come.

There is a Native American proverb that states, "We do not inherit the earth from our ancestors; we borrow it from our children." Using natural, nontoxic skin care products not only helps our skin, it helps us protect what we are borrowing.

SAFE FOR OUR ANIMALS

Creating body care products that are safe for our animal friends means having a commitment to cruelty-free methods of production. The United Kingdom nonprofit organization Research Defence Society (RDS), Understanding Animal Research in Medicine, has estimated that about 50 million animals are used in research worldwide. According to this organization, the United States performs about 15 million procedures on animals each year. Some animal rights organizations feel the number is even higher, claiming that as many as 100 million animals are used in U.S. research each year. Proponents of this type of research argue that animals have played a significant role in advancing medicine. It's true: Without animal research we may not have discovered penicillin, various vaccines, or been able to perfect the process of organ transplants. Few will discount the importance of these and other medical advancements; however, opponents of animal research argue that there are many instances when animal testing is unnecessarily cruel, and I agree with that.

There should be no need for animal testing on products that begin with high-quality, nontoxic ingredients.

The FDA, via the Federal Food, Drug, and Cosmetic Act, does not require the use of animal testing for cosmetic and body care ingredients. And yet, thousands of animals suffer each year.

While most people understand and appreciate the medical breakthroughs made as a result of reasonable and necessary animal testing, I question the necessity of animal testing in the beauty, body care, and household products industries. There should be no need for animal testing on products that begin with high-quality, nontoxic ingredients.

Animal testing refers to an intervention or treatment that can cause the animal pain, fear, and/or suffering and does not provide any benefit to the animal. Some in the scientific community have taken the lead in the area of animal welfare, as it relates to research. More than forty years ago, researchers William Russell, PhD and Rex Burch, PhD, developed the

3 Rs: When possible, *r*eplace animals with alternatives, *r*educe the number of animals used, and *r*efine experiments to include less pain and distress.

"The most humane science is the best science," according to Alan M. Goldberg, PhD, from Johns Hopkins University. "Pain and distress must be eliminated in animal experiments or reduced to an absolute minimum, and, as scientists, we must use the most humane approaches in our research."

As some of those in the scientific community rally around compassionate treatment of research animals, some product manufacturers have become equally concerned. When it comes to beauty and body care, conscientious companies are embracing cruelty-free approaches. Although there is no formal system enforcing the cruelty-free program, manufacturers who use the cruelty-free label commit to using ingredients that were not tested on animals.

It's worth repeating: There is just no need to make animals suffer if the ingredients are nontoxic in the first place. Manufacturers need to take a strong stance on eliminating animal abuse. We can all do our part to end unnecessary animal cruelty. According to the Humane Society of the United States, if more manufacturers of cosmetic, body care, and household products would swear off animal testing, millions of animals would be spared unnecessary pain and suffering.

Even if a consumer of body care and beauty products can set aside the debate about animal compassion, they cannot avoid the obvious: If there is a question as to whether an ingredient may be unsafe for consumers, why use it? Safe, natural, nontoxic ingredients can be used in body care and beauty products. Animal testing in the beauty and body care industries should be a moot point.

Unfortunately, safe, nontoxic ingredients are not the norm. According to a coalition of nonprofit organizations called the Environmental Working Group, every day the average adult uses nine personal care products containing 126 potentially dangerous chemicals. The first step to reduce animal testing is for consumers to read labels carefully and not purchase products that contain toxic ingredients.

According to Karen Lee Stevens, founder and president of All for Animals (www.allforanimals.com), if manufacturers are concerned about safety of their ingredients, there are plenty of alternatives to animal testing. Some of the more common alternatives include cell cultures (also known as in-vitro tests), human volunteers, and database searches of other studies to avoid duplication. The Humane Society reports that alternatives to animal testing can be even more accurate and easier to reproduce. A BBC online report also claims that the stress the animals endure in the labs not only negatively influences the research outcomes, but it can make the results of the experiments meaningless.

Because of the sheer number of beauty and body care products on the market, and the limited number of manufacturers who have a commitment to cruelty-free research and development, it may be difficult to use only cruelty-free products. However, the positive impact that consumers can have on this issue is amazing. According to RDS, a renewed commitment to the 3 Rs by the government of the United Kingdom led to a significant reduction in animal testing.

Choosing cruelty-free beauty and body care products ensures that you are protecting innocent animals. But it can also reinforce your desire to use nontoxic products in the first place.

For a list of cruelty-free companies, visit www.caringconsumer. org and click on "support cruelty-free companies." People for the Ethical Treatment of Animals (www.PETA.org) also provides a list of companies that do not test their products on animals.

THE MEDICINE HORSE STORY

Several years ago, a nonprofit organization in Boulder, Colorado, touched my heart. Over the years, I have tried to support the Humane Society and other "animal friendly" nonprofit organizations, but Medicine Horse was different. I have always loved horses. So, when I heard that Medicine Horse was combining the healing power of horses to help high-risk youth, my curiosity was piqued. As fate would have it, my good friend and coauthor, Karolyn Gazella, is the executive director of this wonderful organization.

According to an article Karolyn wrote for *Elephant* magazine, "Horses epitomize heightened consciousness. Through a keen sense of awareness, the horse can identify and interpret emotions, characteristics, and intention not just in other animals but in people as well. The horse can quickly break down barriers to uncover deep emotions and make room for individual insight."

This work is known as equine-assisted psychotherapy and equine-assisted growth and learning. And it works wonders for young children, especially compared to traditional talk therapy. Medicine Horse has four core programs:

- *Just Say Whoa* helps repeat juvenile offenders;

- *Equus Integration* breaks down barriers among non–English-speaking and English-speaking high school students;

- *Healing With Horses* is a collaboration with hospice that helps young children grieve from a significant loss; and

- *The HopeFoal Project* rescues Premarin foals and matches them with depressed, anxious, and abused teens. I was most drawn to HopeFoal.

Premarin is a widely prescribed hormone-replacement therapy (HRT) drug. *Premarin* actually stands for "PREgnant MAre uRINe." The process is methodical and brutal to the mares. After the mare is impregnated, she is confined to a small pen in which she cannot turn or lay down, a catheter is inserted into her bladder, and the urine is harvested during the last six months of her pregnancy. After giving birth to the foal, the foal is taken away prematurely, the mare is reimpregnated, and the process begins all over again. The quality of life for the mare is horrific. But I was always curious as to what happens to the foal.

To the drug industry, the foals are mere by-products. They don't need the foal, just the mare's urine. Each year, thousands of foals are sent to slaughter and sold to European meat distributors. When the drug was in its heyday, reports indicated that as many as 45,000 foals were slaughtered in just one year. But in 2002, that changed. Why? Not because the drug industry finally realized that it's wrong to kill innocent foals and treat mares in this manner, but because the drug is dangerous.

In response to the Women's Health Initiative (WHI) study, strict warnings were placed on Premarin and the drugs associated with its active ingredients, such as Prempro. Because of the WHI study, and the broad media attention it received, sales of the drug have dropped dramatically. Even after the release of the WHI study, the pharmaceutical industry continues to maintain that the drug is safe and continues to harvest the urine, producing more "by-products" (i.e., foals). Most women don't even know about this "dark side" of the drug they are taking.

In December 2006, news from the M. D. Anderson Cancer Center and the Harbor UCLA Medical Center, presented at the San Antonio Breast Cancer Symposium, linked the reduced usage of hormone-replacement therapy with a steep decline in breast cancer cases. Researchers noted that the most significant decline in breast cancer diagnosis was among women aged fifty to sixty-nine, which coincides with the reduction in hormone-replacement therapy use. According to Francine Grodstein, ScD, associate professor of medicine at Brigham and Women's Hospital in Boston. "It is not news that HT [hormone therapy] increases the risk of breast cancer." While this may not seem "new" to some, researchers agree that this additional information provides even more scientific data as to the direct connection between cancer and Premarin use. And yet, Premarin continues to be a multimillion-dollar drug.

It is not a coincidence that there was a significant decline in breast cancer cases following the dramatically reduced usage of hormone-replacement therapy drugs. There are safer alternatives to these drugs. More important, these alternatives do not come with the heavy price of an innocent foal and a young mare forced to endure such a horrible existence. If you need HRT, ask your doctor about alternatives that do not come from pregnant mare urine.

While hormone therapy is sometimes necessary, using skin care products that contain ingredients which are estrogen mimickers can be dangerous. As mentioned in the previous chapter, toxic ingredients in body care products can actually contribute to estrogen-dependent cancers. We need to avoid chemicals that interfere with our natural hormone balance and cellular communication.

My company, MyChelle Dermaceuticals, is proud to be the corporate sponsor of the Medicine Horse Program HopeFoal Project. In addition, we have spent thousands of dollars in a widespread advertising campaign trying to educate the community about the Premarin industry. And we will never use estrogen disrupters in our products. Never!

I agree with Karolyn as she writes, "For centuries the horse has been a devoted service partner and loyal companion. Today we realize that the horse is also a wise teacher and compassionate healer."

I have often been asked, "Why do you support Medicine Horse when it doesn't have anything to do with skin care?" Philosophically, I believe manufacturers must look beyond their products and give back to the community as a whole. I have chosen to do this by supporting nonprofit organizations like the Medicine Horse Program, the Farm Sanctuary, and the Summit County Animal Shelter. No, they don't have anything to do with skin care, but they have everything to do with helping young teens (and their families) and helping innocent, amazing animals that rely on us. Giving back to such wonderful nonprofit organizations will help improve our world. I have found that consumers who are mindful about their world want to purchase products from mindful manufacturers.

If you would like more information about the Medicine Horse Program, visit the program's website, www.medicinehorse.org. For more information on the Farm Sanctuary, visit www.farmsanctuary.org.

REDEFINING *NATURAL*

The term *natural* has served us well over the years. For me, it defined my way of life and became a professional passion. I realize, however, that the term now needs to be re-defined. Natural ties together a variety of concepts, thoughts, and beliefs. Natural goes beyond merely being present in or produced by nature, as Webster's has described it. The term *natural* should encompass the following key areas:

- Nontoxic and non-estrogenic
- Cruelty-free
- Environmentally safe

Safety is the cornerstone of *natural*. Natural products should be safe for the user and safe for our environment. In the case of body care products, they should also be cruelty-free, making them safe for the animals we share this planet with.

We often see the term *natural*, and its many variations, listed on products. Even if the word *natural* is not used, we often may assume that because there are natural ingredients added, the product is natural. An important lesson I've learned over the years, however, is that just because a product may seem natural doesn't mean it's truly natural and nontoxic. As I have illustrated, many products may contain small amounts of a natural

Natural? You Be the Judge

Here is another label that I found interesting. This product has the word *healing* in its name and the label specifies that it contains white tea. The manufacturer is clearly trying to take advantage of consumers' demand for natural products. Is this product healing or natural? You be the judge.

Water, propylene glycol, cetyl alcohol, fragrance, stearyl alcohol, vitis vinifera (grape) seed oil, ethylhexyl hydroxystearate, clyceryl stearate, palmitic acid, stearic acid, triethanolamine, C12-15 alkyl octanoate, dimethicone, clycerin, carbomer, methyparaben, polysorbate 60, xanthan gum, DMDM hydantoin, propylsorbate 20, camellia sinensis leaf extract, C13-14 isoparaffin, myristic bisabolol, acacia decurrens extract, phenoxyethanol, citrus aurantium amara (bitter orange) flower extract.

Refer back to the last chapter to see how many of these ingredients are actually considered toxic. Remember propylene glycol? When that ingredient goes to the manufacturer, the drum is labeled Avoid Skin Contact because it is so toxic. And yet, it is the second ingredient listed on the label. While the manufacturer made an attempt to add some herbs, it's hard to ignore the toxic chemicals this product contains, like DMDM, parabens, and many others.

DID YOU KNOW?

Organic food, drink, and ingredients are gaining in popularity. According to
The World of Organic Agriculture 2004 Statistics and Emerging Trends,
there were more than 59 million acres (24 million ha) under organic
management. In 2003, there were more than 12,000 certified organic
farmers in the United States.

ingredient but they are far from being natural and nontoxic. This is a
troubling trend. A closer look at these products reveals that they contain
the same old toxic ingredients, just a little added natural twist to confuse
consumers.

Consumers can help redefine *natural* by demanding and using only
nontoxic products. Look beyond the marketing hook when evaluating the
products you use. Avoid products that contain toxic ingredients.

Another Misleading Claim

Have you ever wondered what it means when a cosmetic product label
says DERMATOLOGIST RECOMMENDED? I have. After doing a little research, I
found that there is no governing body that monitors this claim. In fact, it
really has no meaning at all. A manufacturer could have as many as 1 million dermatologists or as few as one who recommend their product—
they can still make that claim. There are also no guidelines that dictate
whether the dermatologist who recommends the product is getting paid
to make the recommendation. There are also no requirements as to how
the dermatologist tested the product so we don't know what the doctor's
recommendation is based on. So, if you're thinking about buying a product because it is DERMATOLOGIST RECOMMENDED, think again. According to
the magazine *Cosmetics & Toiletries*, consumers can get all the information they need from the ingredient listing on the product, rather than
banking on a potentially misleading claim.

In the next chapter, I will take a closer look at that age-old myth that something natural can't be effective and vice versa, that something effective can't be natural.

Along the Journey

Not Natural in New York

I was a guest on a radio program in New York City not that long ago. It was a live call-in show. I just love that format because I get to talk to people from all over the United States. On this particular show, I encountered an irate listener. For the entire first part of the show, the host and I had been talking about the benefits of natural skin care because that's my area of expertise. The host opened up the phone lines and took a call from a woman who was very direct and got straight to the point.

"I don't agree with your guest," the caller said.

"What do you mean?" inquired the host.

"Your guest claims that natural skin care products are the best and I can tell you firsthand that that's just not true. I was having some problems with my skin so I switched to natural products and I am still having the same problems. Just because something claims to be natural, doesn't mean it's better, more effective, or that it will work. It didn't in my case."

It was my turn. "I actually agree with you completely," I said. "Just because a product is called *natural* or it has a few natural ingredients doesn't mean it's a good product." The caller was silent and let me continue.

I explained that the term *natural* has become trite and overused and no longer holds as much meaning as it once did. "I really should correct my terminology," I admitted. "In addition to using the term *natural,* I should also be saying *nontoxic.*"

I explained that, in my view, the two terms—*natural* and *nontoxic*—are synonymous and that many mainstream manufacturers are taking advantage of consumers by making claims and positioning their products as natural when, in fact, they are not. My exchange with the caller continued for a few minutes and then she calmed down.

"Can you go get the products you are presently using?" I asked. She did. "Let's just look at your moisturizer, which is perhaps one of the most important products you can use on your face. What are the ingredients in that natural product?"

"Well, I can't pronounce these things!" she exclaimed in frustration. As it turned out, she wasn't using a natural or nontoxic product at all. She was the victim of a common trend. She was lured by a few vitamins and herbs listed on the front of the package. She was too intimidated to even turn the product around. Once she did, she discovered the truth.

This woman is not alone. I have encountered many people who have an axe to grind with so-called natural products. It's unfortunate, but it's our reality. *Natural* is no longer good enough. We need both natural and nontoxic.

The Solution

4

In the first chapter I gave you an overview of the skin. In this chapter, I'd like to delve a little more deeply into the science of the skin as it relates to bioactive skin care ingredients. Understanding the skin from a scientific perspective helps us understand how we can achieve both safe and effective results from cutting-edge technology and nontoxic ingredients.

There is a widespread misconception that if a product is natural, it is not effective—that it's not strong enough to do the job. Conversely, some people feel that if a product is effective, it can't be natural—that it's more of a drug than a natural product. Research demonstrates that not only are many natural and nontoxic ingredients safe, they can also be very effective. In most cases, these ingredients are even more effective than toxic chemicals. Typically, chemical ingredients are chosen merely because they are cheaper than the natural, nontoxic alternatives. The fact is, we don't need drugs to keep our skin looking and feeling healthy. Nature, when combined with the best science has to offer, can provide us with everything we need.

The key to natural, effective skin care is to find safe products that have a strong scientific foundation. When we access the best of both worlds, we can learn a great deal from both the natural health and the cosmeceutical/dermaceutical industry. Active ingredients can still be natural and safe, and safe and natural ingredients can be active.

DEFINING *DERMACEUTICAL*

More than fifteen years ago, a respected dermatologist, researcher, and professor named Albert M. Kligman, MD, PhD, coined the term *cosmeceutical*. He needed a way to describe the discovery of retinoic acid. To Dr. Kligman, it wasn't appropriate to call retinoic acid a cosmetic ingredient because it has pharmacological, therapeutic properties. According to the research, retinoic acid may help diminish small wrinkles, support collagen formation, and improve the skin's complexion. According to the book *Cosmeceuticals: Active Skin Treatment*, ingredients like retinoic acid achieve cosmetic results via some degree of physiological action. The book lists fruit acids, vitamin E, and hyaluronic acid as other examples of cosmeceuticals.

The definition of a cosmetic is something that beautifies or corrects imperfections. A cosmetic is not considered therapeutic. Dr. Kligman was looking for a descriptive term that went "well beyond the traditional view of cosmetics for merely decorative or camouflage purposes." He wanted to describe ingredients that "do something useful and beneficial."

"Cosmeceuticals are topical cosmetic-pharmaceutical hybrids intended to enhance beauty through ingredients that provide additional health-related function or benefit," according to a report in the *Indian Journal of Pharmacology*. "They are applied topically as cosmetics, but contain ingredients that influence the skin's biological function."

Controversy still surrounds this new term and the cosmeceutical industry in general. However, Dr. Kligman and others have made a significant contribution to the body care industry by recognizing the need for innovation. They revealed how effectively science and nature can work in combination. They came up with the concept of bioactive ingredients. In Dr. Kligman's view, these ingredients and products are designed to meet the needs of an aging population. Baby boomers have become comfortable with the idea of incorporating technological advances into their daily routines. Why not into their body care products?

Even though the Food, Drug, and Cosmetic Act defines cosmetics as "articles intended to be rubbed, poured, sprinkled, or sprayed on, introduced into, or otherwise applied to the human body for cleansing, beautifying, promoting attractiveness, or alteringing the appearance," most people still think of cosmetics as perfumes, lipsticks, mascara, and makeup. There is now a need for a term that is broader than *cosmeceutical*, a term that can be used to describe the entire body care industry, not just cosmetics. That term is *dermaceutical*. *Dermaceutical* describes skin pharmacology. For the purposes of this book, the term *dermaceutical* refers to nontoxic pharmaceuticals for your entire body. I have embraced this term because it takes the

> **DID YOU KNOW?**
>
> *Quality dermaceuticals are built on a foundation of nontoxic bioactives.*

cosmeceutical concept one step further by focusing not just on effective, active pharmacological ingredients, but also on ensuring that those bioactive ingredients are safe and nontoxic. Quality dermaceuticals are built on a foundation of nontoxic bioactives.

BIOACTIVITY BASICS

Our scientific knowledge of the skin and how it functions has increased dramatically in recent years. As discussed in Chapter 1, the outermost layer of the skin is the epidermis. Even though this layer is made up primarily of flat, dead skin cells, we now know that there are finer structures within this layer that are very active. In fact, some components of the epidermis are not dead at all. There is an intricate interaction between the cells in the outermost layer and the growing and more lively cells located in the deeper layers of the skin. In addition, the outer layer controls the appearance and color of the skin, enhances skin strength, and helps activate important enzymes.

"No longer do we have strict differentiation between the dead, upper layer and the living, deeper layers," concludes *Cosmeceuticals: Active Skin Treatment*. This is a significant discovery. If our outermost skin cells are somehow communicating with and influencing our growing basal cells, then we can impact the health of our skin on a deeper level by applying active products to the outermost layer. In addition, if we choose our ingredients wisely and have them at the right dosage and concentration, we can penetrate all layers of the skin, creating vital physiological effects on the health and development of our skin. Conversely, that's also why it's so important to avoid toxic chemical ingredients.

According to Dr. Sabarinathan Kuttalingam Gopalasubramaniam (known as "Dr. K. G."), a scientist who specializes in searching out unique nontoxic ingredients, "A bioactive ingredient produces results. Bioactive ingredients are also recognized and readily received by the skin." To read my interview with Dr. K. G., see page 67.

Just as a toxic chemical can negatively affect the skin, an effective bioactive ingredient positively influences skin cells. As mentioned previously, our skin is often used to deliver some key pharmaceutical agents. Examples of this kind of delivery system include birth control, hormone replacement, and nicotine patches. This application is known as *transdermal*, which literally means "through the skin."

If the pharmaceutical industry can use the skin to deliver drugs, why can't we use the skin to deliver active nutrients and ingredients to help our skin heal and thrive? As it turns out, we can.

In the last two chapters, I have focused on the negative biological effects of toxic ingredients found in many body care products. Now it's time to spotlight proven bioactive skin care ingredients that can positively affect the health of our skin. Bioactive ingredients, applied to the skin, use advanced scientific techniques to maximize the therapeutic activity of these nontoxic, balancing, and rejuvenating substances.

CUTTING-EDGE SKIN CARE

At some point, we have all learned that valuable lesson: If you continue to do the same thing, you'll get the same results. It was Albert Einstein who said that the definition of insanity was doing the same thing over and over again and expecting different results. In skin care, we need to stop doing the same thing over and over again. Stop putting the same cheap, toxic ingredients on our skin. Stop using artificial colorings and fragrances when the natural alternatives look and smell better anyway. Stop ignoring cutting-edge technology. And stop thinking of our skin as an inanimate object rather than the living, complex organ that it is.

I saw a T-shirt the other day with a picture of a television set. Underneath the TV set, it read THINK OUTSIDE THE BOX. That simple phrase has become the mantra for many successful companies. Thinking outside the box is crucial in many aspects of our lives, but it is especially important in the area of innovative skin care.

Skin care has become fully entrenched in a rut—old-school thinking that does not lead to growth, change, and the development of safer and more effective products. Manufacturers are complacent and content to use the same old toxic ingredients. The extent of their innovation is to add minute amounts of a common natural ingredient and label it NEW AND IMPROVED. It's not new and it certainly is not improved. If large cosmetic or skin care manufacturers do invest in research, they are looking for ways to make their product cheaper, last longer on the shelves, or look better. The issue of nontoxic effectiveness is not even on their radar.

In the area of natural, nontoxic dermaceuticals, however, there is a lot going on. I am a curious person by nature. If I hear about an interesting ingredient or read about an exciting new clinical trial involving skin care, it piques my interest right away: I want to learn more about it. I consider myself part business owner and part skin detective. The most exciting and fun part of my job is in the area of research and development. I really enjoy connecting with the scientists and organizations that are making new discoveries.

As a result of my research and discussions with skin care researchers and specialists throughout the world, I've developed my top six list of innovative skin care solutions. In each of these cases, cutting-edge technology, solid science, and proven research methods are utilized to help move the field of natural, nontoxic dermaceuticals forward. Here are six categories I'm most excited about.

1. **Peptides.** A peptide is a protein fraction and a polypeptide is a longer protein chain. Laboratory research has revealed that polypeptides and peptides are biological agents that help slow aging and/or repair damaged skin. Peptides have been shown to stimulate skin regeneration and repair. Examples of important nontoxic skin peptides include the following:

   - Palmitoyl tripeptide-5 (SYN-COLL): a peptide capable of stimulating collagen synthesis in human skin cells.

   - Thymulen 4: induces an increase in the synthesis of keratins (strong proteins) and keratohyalins (a substance in the granular layer of the epidermis).

   - Pisum sativum (Proteasyl TP): a pea peptide that supports and encourages collagen production.

   - AC DermaPeptide Revitalizing: derived from rice, this helps with cellular proliferation, regeneration, and moisturizing.

   - AC DermaPeptide MicroC: derived from cayenne pepper, this peptide increases collagen synthesis and circulation, and works as an anti-irritant.

   - Eyeseryl: has anti-edema properties (that is, it reduces fluid retention) and has been shown to be effective in reducing puffy eyes.

2. **Concentrations that match research studies.** Over the past two decades I have seen product manufacturers make claims for their product ingredients based on scientific studies. Upon further review, I have found that the concentrations in their products don't match the original research. I call this *borrowed science* and it is extremely confusing to the consumer. Cutting-edge technology allows us to research specific ingredients. It's important that the concentrations of those ingredients match those in the studies. A perfect example is the various vitamin C serums now on the market. Researcher Steven S. Traikovich, DO, con-

firms that only the L-ascorbic acid form of vitamin C can be absorbed topically at a concentration of at least 10 percent to enhance collagen production. Subsequent research has confirmed Dr. Traikovich's findings. Obviously, C serums made with less than 10 percent L-ascorbic acid are not consistent with the study results.

3. **Correct form and molecular structure of ingredients.** Technology has taught us that only ingredients with the correct form and molecular structure will be able to penetrate the skin and effect change within the skin's cells. Techniques, such as chiral screening (see page 61 for more information on chirally correct ingredients), ensure that the most absorbable, effective form of each bioactive ingredient is used. In order for an ingredient to be effective, it must be recognized by the skin cells, and have the proper molecular structure to fit the receptor site. It's like opening a door with the correct key; no other key will unlock the door.

4. **Unique plant extracts and marine ingredients.** The world is filled with natural healing substances that are nontoxic, including ingredients from the sea and from plants. The use of rain forest fruits is a great example of the effective collaboration of nature and science. We have learned how to safely and respectfully harvest these amazing therapeutic ingredients in an earth-friendly way. Now we can also use cutting-edge scientific technology to identify the proper concentrations of these important marine and plant nutrients for the skin. For example, the Amazonian fruit camu camu has the highest scientifically documented concentration of vitamin C of any fruit in the world, at more than thirty times that of an orange. Heavy water extracted from the sea, technically known as D_2O, is a prime example of a cutting-edge marine ingredient. D_2O is 100 percent natural and is 10 percent heavier than water. Why is this important? Because heavier water stays on the skin longer and does not evaporate as quickly as typical H_2O. Heavy water also strengthens the skin. Because it has antioxidant activity, heavy water helps protect the skin from external stresses and damage. Other marine ingredients include algae, carrageenan, Venuceane (from deep in the sea of the Gulf of California), Antarctine (from the Antarctic sea),

Abyssine (from deep in the ocean), and marine plankton oligopeptide (a potent sea peptide).

5. **Worldwide discoveries.** Finding natural, nontoxic ingredients means leaving the protective confines of U.S. borders. We are discovering that the most effective and safe natural ingredients actually come from very remote areas of our world. The fruit mangosteen, for example, was originally discovered in the Malay Archipelago, which is a group of islands located between Southeast Asia and Australia. We have learned that mangosteen contains xanthones, which are powerful antioxidants that can heal the skin. Another example is the acai berry from the acai palm tree native to Central and South America, primarily Belize, Brazil, and Peru. This berry contains anthocyanins at a concentration of twenty times that of red wine. These gifts from nature are potent antioxidants that have been researched and can do wonders for our skin.

6. **Ingredient synergy.** Putting ingredients together to maximize their effectiveness is not only based on science, it is an art, requiring a blend of intuition, logic, and insight about the most effective ingredient formulation. The art of formulating effective and safe skin care products begins and ends with the concept of synergy—what works best together. It's similar to putting together that perfect outfit for a special event. What fits together to create the right look? Will the shoes complement the dress? Likewise, when it comes to skin care, some ingredients can enhance the action and complement the strengths of other ingredients. For example, a variety of antioxidants work well together, such as combining L-ascorbic acid and astaxanthin. Both of these antioxidants help ease inflammation, but they do it in different ways. For more information about formulating products, see "The Art of Formulating" on page 61.

These six cutting-edge advances form the bedrock for the development of more effective, safer dermaceutical products. One of the most innovative technological advances in skin care is the use of chirally correct ingredients.

CHIRAL IS CRITICAL

Chiral (pronounced KI-ral) refers to the characteristic of molecules that appear in mirror image form. The famous chemist Louis Pasteur first recognized chirality in his laboratory. The word *chiral* comes from the Greek word *chir*, meaning "hand." Your hands are mirror images of each other, just like your feet and your eyes. If you try to place your left-handed glove on your right hand, it becomes very clear that it was not designed to fit;

The Art of Formulating

Creating nontoxic, effective skin care products requires the perfect combination of science and nature. It truly is an art. It is very important to choose ingredients that complement and enhance each other. According to scientist and ingredient specialist Dr. Sabarinathan K. G., "You don't want the ingredients to work against each other. You want a synergistic blend of supportive ingredients focusing on a specific problem or skin type and you want them to work from different directions."

The amount of each ingredient is carefully calculated. Like a chef in a five-star restaurant, the product formulator decides which ingredients work best together to create a masterpiece. Each ingredient is evaluated for potency, desired therapeutic objective, pH, and synergy. When the product is completed, the end result is an exquisite combination of safety and effectiveness.

Bioactive, nontoxic ingredients have a positive, synergistic effect. In the case of toxic chemicals, there can be a negative, synergistic effect. The interactions of several of these chemicals can combine to create even more toxicity. For example, according to Dr. K. G., use of synthetic vitamin E (dl-alpha tocopherol) in place of the natural version (d-alpha tocopherol) can cause allergic reactions, and those reactions can be complicated and aggravated when combined with other chemicals. "Combining toxic ingredients compounds the potential problem," he explained.

likewise, your right shoe won't fit your left foot. Just like our hands and feet, most molecules are chiral, meaning they exist in left- and right-handed forms. Chiral compounds are involved in every process of the human body. In most cases, these processes require the right-handed or left-handed form of the molecule, but not both, and in some cases they are neutral without a left or right designation.

Chirally correct skin care ingredients fit perfectly into the skin cell's receptor, just as your left-handed glove fits onto your left hand. The skin cells have the ability to determine which ingredients are beneficial, useless, or harmful. Skin cells can easily recognize chirally correct natural ingredients. The cells identify those ingredients as a good fit and something they need. That's why chirally correct ingredients are so effective. Increased absorption is an additional benefit of bioactive, chirally correct ingredients. This is especially beneficial in cases of aged, sun-damaged, acne-prone, or sensitive skin. Normal skin function is compromised in these conditions, so it is crucial for active ingredients to be easily recognized, absorbed, and uti-

Cosmetic Dermatology

I was talking to a friend the other day about her eczema. She told me that she had to find a new dermatologist because her old doctor has decided to switch his entire practice over to cosmetic dermatology. This is a fancy way of saying that he can make more money giving Botox shots and doing laser treatments than offering traditional medical treatment.

According to *Skin & Aging* magazine, there is a widening gap between medical and cosmetic dermatology. The problem, reports contributing editor Louis Pilla, may be leading to a shortage of medical dermatologists. For example, in Winston-Salem, North Carolina, you have to wait as long as ten weeks for an appointment with a medical dermatologist, but the wait is far shorter if you want a Botox treatment. Unfortunately, consumers are paying the price. This shift is forcing people to become more proactive about the health of their skin.

lized by the skin. This helps restore the skin's integrity, reduces inflammation, and enhances the skin's immune function without causing irritation.

The application of this technology results in slightly more expensive product formulations, but the results are well worth it. While chirally correct ingredients are especially beneficial to compromised skin, they are effective for all skin types, including normal functioning skin.

Here are some great examples of chirally correct ingredients:

- **D-alpha tocopherol:** This natural form of vitamin E is a powerful antioxidant, free-radical scavenger, moisturizer, and natural preservative because it protects against oxidation.

- **D-beta fructans:** These are glucose chain molecules from date palms that boost the skin's immunity and build moisture.

- **D-beta glucosamine:** From the Chinese foxglove plant, this has been shown to lead to tighter alignment of the epidermis and dermis.

- **D-boldine:** A potent anti-inflammatory and antioxidant, this comes from the South American boldo plant.

- **D-panthenol:** This part of the water-soluble vitamin B complex (B$_5$) acts as a penetrating moisturizer.

- **L-sodium hyaluronate:** This is the major constituent of collagen production and a powerful humectant that helps the skin hold water, maintain moisture, and prevent dehydration.

- **L-ascorbic acid:** The most effective and stable form of vitamin C and a great antioxidant. To be effective in stimulating collagen, a formulation must contain at least a 10 percent concentration of L-ascorbic acid.

Hyaluronic acid is an excellent example of the effective use of chiral technology. Hyaluronic acid is a key component of the cellular matrix of the dermis, keeping it in tighter alignment with the epidermis. Hyaluronic acid in its large molecular state is not recognized by or beneficial for the skin cells; however, the chiral form, known as L-sodium hyaluronate, is taken up by cells deep within the skin because it mirrors the form of

NONTOXIC ALTERNATIVES

TOXIC INGREDIENT	NONTOXIC ALTERNATIVES
Parabens and other preservatives	Stabil (phenethyl alcohol from rose, bananas, apple, and lily)
	Plantservative (from honeysuckle)
	Sodium hydroxymethylglycinate (from amino acids)
	Enzymes (such as glucose oxidase and lactoperoxidase)
	Olive leaf (olea europaea)
	Oregano (origanum vulgare)
	Tea tree essential oil
	Thyme essential oil
	Grapefruit seed extract
	Bitter orange extract
Synthetic (perfume) fragrances	Essential oils
	Herbal and floral extracts
DEA and other toxic emulsifiers	Plant waxes (such as candelilla, carnuaba, jojoba, and rice bran)
	Xanthan gum
	Quince seed
Propylene glycol and other toxic humectants	Lecithin panthenol (pro-vitamin B_5)
	Zemea propanediol (from corn sugar)
	Glycerin
	Vitamin E
Sulfates (such as sodium lauryl/ laureth sulfate)	Coconut fatty acids
	Yucca saponins
	Amaranth foaming peptide

hyaluronic acid that already exists in the skin. Vitamin C works in a similar fashion. The skin will not gain much benefit by simply applying vitamin C topically. However, when the chiral form, known as L-ascorbic acid, is applied directly to the skin, it has been clinically shown to help the skin maintain collagen production and help keep the skin firm. As mentioned previously, this form of vitamin C matches the clinical studies done on using vitamin C to diminish the look of wrinkles.

If you are looking for nontoxic, extremely effective skin care products, look for ingredients listed on page 64.

OTHER MUST-HAVE INGREDIENTS

In addition to chirally correct ingredients, there are many other nontoxic ingredients that are true shining stars. For more information on other "must-have" ingredients, I decided to ask for a little help from my good friend, Morag Currin. Morag is the president and founder of Touch for Cancer, a restorative skin care and massage training program for licensed or certified aestheticians and beauty therapists. A native of South Africa, Morag owned her own skin care clinic, created her own Oncology Aesthetic program, and is certified in many spa modalities.

Here are Morag's top five innovative ingredient picks:

1. **Carnisine.** This multifunctional dipeptide is a powerful antioxidant specific to the skin. This is especially important as we age because cellular proteins undergo destructive changes as a result of oxidation. Carnisine is effective against many forms of protein modification, which leads to skin cell degradation and accelerated aging.

2. **Myrtle.** This anti-aging ingredient delays cellular senescence (the process of growing old) and limits dermal degeneration (skin aging).

3. **Palmitoyl oligopeptide.** This ingredient stimulates key constituents of the skin and is as effective as retinol against wrinkles, but it does not cause skin irritations.

4. **R-lipoic acid.** This highly bioavailable antioxidant is both water- and fat-soluble, which enables it to penetrate the cellular membrane.

5. **CoQ_{10}.** Also known as ubiquinone or idebenone, this ingredient neutralizes key free radicals and is an excellent antioxidant that works well in high-altitude environments.

In many cases, fruit pulps can be especially healing to the skin. "Many fruit pulps provide enzymatic activity to the outer layer of the skin, simultaneously supporting it with antioxidant properties," explained Morag. The enzymatic activity also helps smooth and revive skin. The wonderful fibrous texture and natural aromatic qualities of fruit pulps are also healing. Fruit pulps have been shown to irritate sensitive skin conditions and should not be used until the skin has been normalized.

CONCLUSION

We have certainly made some significant advances in the area of therapeutic, nontoxic skin care product ingredients. However, this technology and the implementation of these advances have not made it far enough into the mainstream. As a result, many people are still using products that may cause toxic side effects and damage the skin.

There are nontoxic alternatives to the toxic ingredients that remain in many skin care products. In addition, by tapping into the existing scientific technology and cutting-edge information that is available, we can use nontoxic ingredients that are also therapeutically effective. The scientific literature demonstrates that these bioactive ingredients provide significant benefits and can give consumers the results they deserve. Using these active ingredients to create quality, nontoxic dermaceutical products is the way of the future.

"The future promises increasingly sophisticated formulations for cosmetics and skin care products," according to a 2005 article in the *Indian Journal of Pharmacology*. "The trend towards therapeutic cosmetics is sure to result in the need to obtain a better understanding of modern ingredients and assessment techniques," the authors conclude.

We can apply the best of both worlds to skin care: adopting the best that nature has to offer, while taking advantage of appropriate technological advances. Now that you know what ingredients to look for, it's time to help you customize your skin care regimen.

Along the Journey

Corresponding with a Scientist

Over the years I have had many opportunities to talk to scientists, tour labs and manufacturing facilities, and ask a lot of questions. Keeping on top of research and development in this way is one of the things I love most about skin care. It's exciting for me to learn new things.

One of the more interesting scientists I have corresponded with is Sabarinathan Kuttalingam Gopalasubramaniam, PhD. For obvious reasons, he does not mind being called Dr. K. G. Dr. K. G.'s specialty is searching out unique and effective ingredients. He is a fellow with the University of Autonomous De Morelos in Mexico, but he spends most of his time at the Center of Advanced Studies in Agricultural Microbiology at Tamil Nadu Agricultural University in India. Because of Dr. K. G.'s specialty, I sought him out to learn more about bioactives. Here is an excerpt of our correspondence:

Q. What are some of the more innovative skin care ingredients available today?

A. There are many nontoxic, effective ingredients available. State-of-the-art antioxidants with high potency are very innovative. Examples include astaxanthin, which is a thousand times more potent than vitamin E. Resveratrol from wine and other sources has anti-aging effects and is great for the skin. PBN, also known as a Spin Trap ingredient, helps trap harmful free radicals and prevents them from damaging skin cells. D-beta glucosamine is an antioxidant that helps the skin's immune support cells.

In addition to antioxidants, there are many others, including D_2O, or heavy water, which is a unique "moisture" form of water. Totarol, from the totara tree in New Zealand is antibacterial and will help acne. D-beta fructan is an herb that helps moisture-starved skin, just as it helps plants during a drought. L-sodium hyaluronate helps skin retain water and stay plumped. Amino-guanidine—from turnip juice, mushrooms, corn germ, and rice hulls—helps prevent wrinkles and is a great antioxidant.

Q. That's pretty impressive. From a technology standpoint, what do you
see as significant advances?

A. The advent of chirally correct ingredients is significant. This is when the
molecular structure of an ingredient that is grown in the lab mirrors what is
grown in nature. Selecting natural ingredients—whether directly from the
earth or from a controlled source in the lab—is critical. Unfortunately, many
companies do not pay attention to this.

Mixing technology has also been advancing. We now know that when we
mix smaller batches with less heat, we can keep the active ingredients active.

Q. Are there alternatives to the toxic ingredients that are presently being
used in many skin care products?

A. Absolutely. There are many advances in this area. There are nontoxic preservatives and emulsifiers available. For fragrances, a blend of essential oils and
extracts can be used. As I mentioned earlier, it's unfortunate that many companies do not focus on this.

Q. How significant is it to have bioactive ingredients in skin care products?

A. It's very significant if you want to produce results. Where there is activity,
there is potential for change. No activity equals no results.

Consumers need to be aware of ingredients that can make a product effective. Just because a product is nontoxic doesn't mean it has any real benefit.
There may be just a fairy dusting of key active ingredients, but basically the
product is still useless. Today, we can produce products that are not only nontoxic but go much further by using sophisticated, targeted ingredients in levels
that are strong enough to make a positive change in the skin.

5

Determine
Your Skin Type

*O*ur world is filled with all kinds of people—unique individuals each with their own personalities and attributes. We are all physically, emotionally, and biochemically different. It is our individuality that makes life interesting, and at times, complex. The same is true with skin care.

You've probably heard someone say, "Oh, I know the type." They are most likely referring to a personality type. The problem with skin care is that we often *don't* know the "type." To be more specific, we don't truly understand our own skin type. The type of skin we have can add a level of complexity to our skin care routine. This is especially true with the skin on our face. As experts have learned more about the skin, they have also discovered that understanding skin type is critical.

Individualizing your skin care routine for optimal effectiveness begins with determining your skin type. "Some women are quite aware of their skin type; for other women, it's a complete mystery, an elusive conundrum of changes that never settles down in one specific direction," according to Paula Begoun, author of *The Beauty Bible*. "Skin type strongly influences our decisions about our skin care routines."

Identifying and understanding your skin type will help you optimize your skin care routine. In the long run, it will also save you money because you will be able to buy products that will actually be effective, rather than products that just sit on your shelves because they don't work or, even worse, cause irritation.

ONE SIZE DOES *NOT* FIT ALL

In the previous chapters I discussed what ingredients can be toxic to the skin and what ingredients are healing and therapeutic for the skin. But what makes skin care so exciting, is determining which ingredients should be used safely and effectively for a specific skin type. To have healthy, vibrant skin, we first need to know what we are dealing with. Because there are different types of skin, there are also different skin care regimens. When it comes to skin care, an individualized approach is the most effective.

There are a variety of external and internal factors that influence our skin type. Some of these can be controlled and some cannot. It is important to be aware of all the factors that can contribute to your skin type and the health of your skin so you can positively influence your skin's health whenever possible.

Targeted, well-formulated skin care products balance the deficiencies in specific skin types, focusing on the health of the skin. That's why it is so critical to properly identify your skin type. Solving the skin type mystery requires careful inspection of all the clues. Let's take a closer look at issues that can help determine your skin type.

Hormonal Changes

Hormones are powerful chemical substances produced by endocrine glands. Endocrine glands include:

- the ovaries (testes in men)
- the pituitary and pineal glands, in the brain
- the thyroid and parathyroid, in the neck
- the pancreas, behind the stomach
- the thymus, in the chest
- the adrenals, on top of each kidney

Hormones are powerful chemical messengers that influence physiological functions and interact with other key body systems. Hormonal activity is very complex. Volumes could be written on this topic alone.

However, for the purpose of skin health, we know that as our hormones fluctuate, our skin—and our skin type—can change. Significant hormonal changes can occur during extreme stress, puberty, menstruation, pregnancy, perimenopause, and menopause. For example, when I was pregnant with my daughter, my skin became hyperpigmented (varying degrees of dark- and light-colored skin).

Climate and Weather

The climate where you live can influence your skin dramatically. Your skin will be affected if the weather is hot, cold, dry, damp, or humid. Moving to a new climate or elevation may also change your skin type. Where I live in the Rocky Mountains the climate is very dry. After moving to Colorado, I needed to change my hydrating routine dramatically. My skin type changed from normal/acne to dehydrated/acne practically overnight. The same is true if you move from a dry to a moist climate. If you travel a lot, the weather will affect your skin. And, of course, extremely cold climates can be hard on the skin, causing lack of oil production and dehydration. Sunny, warm climates can dramatically affect skin type by increasing the oil production in the skin. The climate you live in should always be considered when evaluating your skin type.

Sun Exposure

Sunlight influences your skin type throughout your entire life. Be aware that there is no such thing as a "healthy tan." For decades, people have been told that if you have a tan, you look healthy. In addition, having a tan was a status symbol; it indicated that you were vacationing in tropical resorts and enjoying a life of privilege. Today most of us understand the damaging effects of unprotected sun exposure. Wearing wide-brimmed hats and sitting in shaded areas by the pool or on the beach has become in vogue. I have found, however, that it is sometimes nearly impossible to find a place in the shade. I have learned to pack a beach umbrella to stick in the sand so I can protect myself and my family from the sun. Keep in mind that if you were exposed to unprotected sunlight as a child, your skin type as an adult will be influenced by that previous exposure, even if you don't spend a lot of time in the sun now. Because sunlight is one of the most influential factors associated with skin type and the health of our skin, I've devoted an entire chapter to the topic (Chapter 7). The bottom line when it comes to sun exposure is that sunlight is a major cause of aging skin, hyperpigmentation (dark skin patches), and cancer. Protecting your skin from the sun is critical, no matter what your skin type. The sun is public enemy number one in the fight against premature aging and skin cancer.

Health Problems and Medications

Skin conditions, such as rosacea (discussed later in this chapter), psoriasis, and eczema, hyper- or hypothyroid conditions, and cancer can also influence your skin type. If you are on prescription medications, your skin type may change. Some medications that can affect your skin include birth control pills, hormone replacement and cholesterol-lowering drugs, and acne treatments. Some prescription drugs can also make your skin more sensitive to the sun. If you are taking prescription medications, ask your physician or pharmacist if they can influence your skin in any way.

Skin Care Products

Using the wrong nourishing cream, overexfoliating, or using products that contain toxic ingredients will definitely affect your skin type. Your skin care routine and the products you use daily can change your skin type—for better or worse. Some ingredients can dry the skin and some chemicals can create sensitive skin. Be very careful about the products you use on your skin. For more specific information on toxic and nontoxic ingredients, see Chapters 2 and 4.

Diet and Lifestyle

What you eat and what you do dramatically affects your skin type. Smoking, for example, is very detrimental to the skin. Smoking hampers circulation and therefore deprives the skin of vital nutrients and oxygen, which can lead to a gray and lifeless complexion. Exercise can positively influence your skin. Your skin type may change if you are exercising on a regular basis. A low-fat diet can cause skin to become dry, while a diet high in trans fats can cause excessive oil production. For more information about diet and lifestyle factors that influence the skin, see Chapter 9.

Genetics

Your genes can also influence your skin type. For example, if your mother had oily skin, you may have a genetic predisposition to oily skin. Remember, however, that genetics is just one factor and genetics only gives you a predisposition to a particular skin type. A predisposition is far different than an inevitability. If possible, find out your parents' skin type. Remember, the goal is to gather as much information you can to accurately determine your own skin type.

Skin type myth: You will always have the same skin type.

These factors interact to influence your skin type. Just as there is no single skin type, there is no single reason why you have a certain skin type. Many variables work together to create your skin type. The most significant thing to keep in mind is that your skin changes continually. Remember, your skin is a living organ. As discussed in Chapter 1, depending on your age, the life cycle of a skin cell can be less than a month, so it makes sense that your skin type will change. In fact, you can bet on it!

Skin type reality: Your skin type will fluctuate frequently based on your body's hormonal activity, the weather, stress in your life, your diet, and many other factors.

Be vigilant about your skin type. Just as your skin adapts to your internal and external environment, you may need to adapt your skin care routine to your changing skin type. The first step, of course, is to learn more about each of the skin type categories. Don't try to determine your skin type after it has been freshly washed or while you have makeup on. To conclusively identify your skin type, you may also want to gain input from a professional.

NORMAL SKIN

Normal is one of those subjective terms that can be interpreted in many different ways. When it comes to skin types, *normal* refers to skin that is in proper balance. According to *Modern Esthetics: A Scientific Source for Estheticians*, your skin is normal when "the glands produce just the right amount of sebum and sweat. . . . It has a soft, smooth texture and is clear." Typically, people with normal skin have very few issues with their skin, other than an occasional or minor breakout during menstruation or high-stress times. Normal skin also does not show any unusual sensitivity. People with normal skin have no signs of oily or dry zones.

Normal skin is very rare. Nearly everyone has slightly sensitive skin or some areas that are dehydrated, hyperpigmented, and/or clogged with white- or blackheads.

The skin care routine for people with normal skin includes cleansing and then using a nourishing cream in the morning and evening. An exfoliating fruit peel once a week and an enzyme scrub is recommended to assist in skin tissue respiration. This will also enhance the penetration of the nutrients applied in serums and nourishing creams.

OILY SKIN

With oily skin, the skin is out of balance because the sebaceous (oil) glands are producing more oil than is needed. As a result, the skin is shiny and may feel greasy. The pores are visible and enlarged. Because of the excess oil, the pores are often clogged and there may be a large number of blackheads. Blackheads alone, however, do not indicate that you have oily skin, but there is a strong likelihood that if you have black- or whiteheads, you do have oily skin.

Blackheads could be formed not just by oil deposits but by the oxidation of cosmetic products trapped inside the pores, combined with dead skin cells lingering within the pores due to poor exfoliation. This, in fact, was my problem. To this day, if I do not regularly exfoliate, I tend to get clogged pores, which eventually leads to infected acne lesions. People with oily skin are prone to acne. You may have many blemishes or few blemishes, depending on your skin. Acne is so common because oily skin is one of the most common skin types.

What's challenging about oily skin is that, in some cases, the skin appears dry. This may seem like an oxymoron; however, too much oil production can impair the skin's outer layer. When the pores become clogged, the oil can't make it to the outer layer to lubricate the skin. The skin may appear dry but the cause is excess oil. "And oily skin can lack moisture," explains *Modern Esthetics*, "either because it has been overscrubbed or alcohol-based products have dried it out." Clogged pores are the best indicator of oily skin.

Individuals with oily skin will benefit from using a cleanser that contains cranberry extract, alpha hydroxy acids, and beta hydroxy acids, and a nourishing cream that contains totarol, cranberry extract, and essential oil of lemongrass. Cranberry, totarol, horopito, and essential oil of lemongrass have antibacterial and/or anti-inflammatory properties. Lemongrass can also help balance oil production. A fruit-based peel or mud mask with bentonite and kaolin should be used once or twice a week, depending on the severity of the condition. People with oily skin will also benefit from an oil-controlling serum daily. For more information on effective acne treatment, see the next chapter.

DRY SKIN

Dry skin has no noticeable oily zones. The skin is thin and feels dry and rough. Pores are very small and, in some cases of extreme dryness, pores are nearly invisible. People with dry skin often also have a pale or light complexion. Flaking is characteristic of this skin type, and the skin may even feel tight because it is so dry. Some people with dry skin may also have some degree of skin sensitivity.

Dryness results when skin cannot adequately retain moisture. Sensitivity results when there is a lack of moisture and oil is out of balance, permitting the entry of outside irritants.

Climate, lifestyle factors, and diet can all contribute to dry skin. Nutritional deficiencies can weaken your skin's ability to repair and rebuild itself. Skin will also become drier as it ages, due to decreased hormonal activity.

Products for dry skin should contain ingredients that not only hydrate the skin but also keep moisture locked in. Cactus flower extract, antarcticene, and peptides are examples of ingredients that will leave the skin feeling dewy and moist. Other hydrating ingredients include D-ceramides, cassia beta-glycan, D-beta fructan, squalane (from Spanish olives), rosehip seed oil, pomegranate seed oil, cloudberry seed oil, and L-sodium hyaluronate.

COMBINATION SKIN

Just as the term indicates, combination skin is a combination of oily and dry areas. The focus here should be on normalizing the skin by balancing moisture retention and oil production.

People with the most common type of combination skin have oily skin

SKIN TYPE INGREDIENTS

	ACNE/OILY	DRY	SENSITIVE	MATURE
M U S T H A V E	totarol	heavy water	heavy water	Thymulen 4
	retinol	D-beta fructan	EGF	marine oligopeptide
	salicylic acid 2%	rose hips seed oil	kombucha	SYN-COLL
	horopito	D-beta glucosamine	coconut milk/fat	SYN-TACKS
	glycolic acid polymer 1%	squalane		L-sodium hyaluronate
	cranberry extract	sphingolipids		L-ascorbic acid
	essential oil of lemongrass	phospholipids		Venuceane
		NaPCA (L-sodium PCA)		copper peptide
		cassia beta-glycans		L-proline
		L-sodium hyaluronate		
H E L P F U L	stone root extract	PBN	sea buckthorn	NaPCA (L-Sodium PCA)
	hamamelis extract	Thymulen 4	passionflower	
	D-biotin			L-superoxide dismutase
	L-limonene			cassia beta-glycans
				cloudberry

in the T-zone (the forehead, nose, and chin) and dry skin everywhere else. The degree of both oiliness and dryness varies on a case-by-case basis.

To treat combination skin, it is important to use products designed to support balanced oil production and hydrate the entire face. Even the most oily skin can be dehydrated. If the skin is adequately hydrated, it can detoxify on its own more efficiently. We need to support the skin's natural functions.

SENSITIVE SKIN

When the outer layer of the skin is impaired, it can become sensitive to outside irritants, as well as a variety of product ingredients. According to Leslie Bauman, MD, 40 percent of Americans report that they have sensitive skin. Symptoms of sensitive skin may include redness, itching, stinging, or burning. There may also be visible surface veins. Many individuals with this skin type are also prone to allergic reactions. Sensitive skin is thin

SKIN TYPE INGREDIENTS

	Rosacea	Exfoliation	Puffy Eyes and Dark Circles
MUST HAVE	willow herb extract totarol folic acid vitamin B_{12} kombucha	super concentrated pumpkin extract honey enzymes pumpkin enzymes AHA BHA glycolic acid polymer 1%	eyeseryl daisy
HELPFUL	heavy water turmeric	retinol	

and fine-textured and can react quickly to cold and heat. As a result, people with sensitive skin are also prone to windburn and sunburn.

If you have sensitive skin, test a new product on a small part of your skin before using it liberally. People with sensitive skin need to be vigilant about the ingredients in their products—more than the average individual. Even natural fruit pulps and peels should be avoided until the skin becomes more balanced. Even though these wonderful exfoliating pulps provide antioxidant nutrition for the skin, they can sting sensitive skin.

Sensitive skin that is inflamed will benefit from ingredients such as squalane (from Spanish olives), kombuchka, L-sodium hyaluronate, willow, arnica, licorice, and gotu kola. Using a hydrating mist throughout the day will help ease inflammation and keep the skin hydrated. Be sure the mist contains heavy water, turmeric, D-beta fructan, and D-beta glucosamine from Chinese foxglove.

MATURE SKIN

According to a 2007 report by Metropolitan Life, 26 percent of the population is over age forty-three. In fact, there are more than 40 million baby boomers over the age of fifty. That means there are a lot of people who fall into the *mature skin* category. Mature skin is typically lacking in oil and moisture and can sometimes be dry. You may see superficial lines, as well as deepening expression lines—those dreaded wrinkles—in mature skin.

DID YOU KNOW?

Long-term stress is a major factor in premature aging. Stress causes your adrenal glands to secrete stress hormones, responsible for causing dry and/or oily patches, acne, and, in severe cases, limiting the supply of blood flowing to the skin, resulting in dull, lifeless skin. In addition to making you secrete stress hormones, stress creates free radicals that attack healthy living cells, including skin cells.

What About Ethnic Skin?

Individuality is a big part of successful skin care, and our ethnicity is a big part of our individuality. Very few studies evaluating the effects of ethnicity on skin care have been conducted. As a result, we don't know precisely how ethnicity affects skin type. We do know that ethnicity directly affects the pigment content of the skin and could explain why fair-skinned people are more prone to skin cancer than people of color. A study published in the *American Journal of Clinical Dermatology* found that water loss is greater among people who have black skin and that these individuals have a lower water content. This could indicate that a focus on hydration is important for people who belong to certain ethnic populations. Researchers whose work was featured in the *Journal of the American Academy of Dermatology* concluded, "There is not a wealth of data on racial and ethnic differences in skin and hair structure, physiology, and function. What studies do exist involve small patient populations and often have methodological flaws. Consequently, few definitive conclusions can be made."

There is a loss of elasticity, especially around the eyes. Because of the loss of elasticity, the skin may also sag around the eyes, cheeks, and throat. The skin may also become sensitive because it's so fragile.

This is such an important topic, I devoted an entire chapter to age-defying skin care. For more information on caring for mature skin and preventing some of the symptoms associated with mature skin, see Chapter 8.

Keep in mind, that age is not the sole indicator of mature skin. You may only be thirty-five years old chronologically, but your total sun exposure, lifestyle, stress, party habits, and past use of toxic skin care products, can add up to ten years to your skin. This kind of abuse will always be first evident in the skin on your face. The good news is that if we take care of our bodies and skin, we can look good at any age and even reverse the visible signs of aging.

Another skin condition that some baby boomers are faced with is the development of rosacea.

ROSACEA

According to www.rosacea.org, rosacea (pronounced roh-ZAY-sha) is more common than people think, mostly because the baby boom generation is entering the most susceptible ages. An estimated 14 million Americans have rosacea. What's worse, many of them may not even realize they have it. A Gallup survey found that 78 percent of Americans don't know what rosacea is, how to recognize it, or how to treat it.

Rosacea is a skin condition that can first appear as a red rash, primarily on the nose and cheeks. "Most people expect to leave facial skin problems behind when they reach adulthood, so they're often puzzled and frustrated by the onset of rosacea," John Wolf, MD, chairman of dermatology at Baylor University College of Medicine, told www.rosacea.org. "While the early signs of the disorder may come and go unexpectedly, without treatment it tends to grow more persistent and severe, posing a substantial impact both physically and on people's emotional, social, and professional lives," explained Dr. Wolf.

This condition involves inflammation of the small blood vessels in the capillaries of the face. The red rash is usually symmetrical and intermittent depending on individual triggers. Symptoms of rosacea may include papules (small solid bumps), pustules (inflamed, pus-filled bumps), and/or solid, firm bumps resembling classic acne all over the cheeks and nose. If this condition is left untreated and progresses, a bulbous nose (similar to W. C. Fields's) may develop.

More people ask me about rosacea than I ever thought possible. I have seen the early signs in friends who have a flare-up after a glass of wine or some spicy food. The skin on their face immediately becomes flushed and inflamed. Even moderate exercise or a short time in a steam room or hot tub can bring on symptoms of rosacea.

While there is no known cause or cure for rosacea, researchers from the University of California–San Diego School of Medicine recently found that this condition stems from an overproduction of two interactive inflammatory proteins, which, in turn, causes an excess of a third protein. The reason this discovery is so significant is that conventional medicine currently treats rosacea with antibiotics. "Our findings may modify the therapeutic approach to treating rosacea, since bacteria aren't the right target," concluded research team leader Richard L. Gallo, MD. According to Dr. Gallo, antibiotics have helped to some degree with mild symptom relief because some of them inhibit the inflammatory enzymes; however, long-term antibiotic use may be detrimental.

Proper diagnosis of rosacea is important. If you have rosacea, avoid products with irritating, toxic ingredients. Your focus should be on products that contain ingredients to help control and treat inflamed, irritated skin. Anti-inflammatory herbal ingredients include totarol, willow, arnica, chamomile, and essential oil of blue chamomile. You should also use a nourishing cream that supports the skin's internal structure and integrity. From a dietary and lifestyle standpoint, I recommend the following:

- Take a comprehensive antioxidant and multivitamin supplement daily.
- Exercise in moderation.
- Avoid spicy foods.
- Limit alcohol consumption.
- Do not smoke.
- Avoid direct sun exposure, especially on the face.

If you have any of the following warning signs, see a dermatologist to obtain a proper diagnosis:

- redness on the cheeks, nose, chin, or forehead
- small visible blood vessels on the face
- bumps or pimples on the face
- watery or irritated eyes

Rosacea can be a chronic and complex skin disorder. As with many conditions, if it is caught early, it can be managed successfully.

OUR CHANGING SKIN

As the old saying goes, the only constant in life is change. This is true of skin types as well. As I mentioned previously, I live in the beautiful Colorado Rocky Mountains. When I first moved to Colorado, I heard someone say, "If you don't like the weather, just wait fifteen minutes, because it will change." Predicting skin type can be just as unpredictable as predicting the weather. It can change with the seasons, the time of month, and even the time of day (especially those extremely stressful days!).

No matter what your skin type, you need to consider a variety of factors, including the overall health of your skin, your skin's condition, and the function/benefit of product ingredients. The best way to avoid irritation, no matter what your skin type, is to use products that contain nontoxic ingredients. Alternatives to many of the toxic ingredients on the market today are featured in the chart on page 64 in Chapter 4.

There are times when skin care goes beyond a particular type. Sometimes there can be a skin challenge that deserves special attention. Acne is a prime example, and it's discussed in detail in the next chapter.

SKIN TYPE	CHARACTERISTICS	
Normal/Balanced	Soft, smooth texture	Very few, if any, blemishes
	Pores not clearly visible	Even tone and color
Oily	Thick, greasy texture	Pores enlarged and clogged
	Tends to be shiny	Considerable number of black- and/or whiteheads
Dry	Dull, pale appearance	Pores small or almost invisible
	Fine, thin texture	May be considerable flaking and fine lines
	Feels dry and rough	
Combination	Oily in the T-zone common	Dehydrated in some areas
	Blemishes confined to one or two areas	
Sensitive	Red, itchy, burning, or stinging	Thin in texture
	Prone to allergic reactions	Prone to windburn and sunburn
Mature	Loss of elasticity	May be dry and/or sensitive
	Superficial and/or deepening lines (wrinkles)	

The T-Zone

Oftentimes, parts of the face are referred to as *zones*. The most notable zone is the T-zone. The T-zone refers to the area of the face on the forehead (the top of the T), down the nose, and on the chin. Problems can occur in the T-zone because there are more oil glands there. As a result, those areas may be oilier and tend to break out more than other parts of the face. When the T-zone is oily but the rest of the face is dry or normal, this is known as the complex skin type called *combination*. No matter what skin type you have now, combination skin will surface at some point in your life, if it hasn't already. When evaluating your skin type, remember to pay close attention to your T-zone.

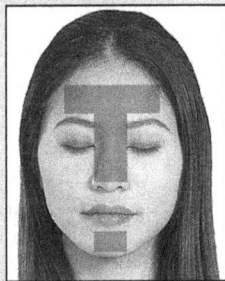

Along the Journey

I Know My Type . . .

I travel a lot. As a result, I meet many new people while sitting on the runway waiting for takeoff. I remember a particularly friendly woman I met on a flight from Chicago back to Colorado. I had just given a seminar on nontoxic, effective skin care.

After we settled into our seats, we asked each other the typical introductory questions. "What do you do for a living?" she asked on cue. When I told her about my company, she was visibly excited. This woman wanted to talk about her skin. She was in her mid-forties and I could tell that she had dry skin.

"I have really sensitive skin," she proceeded. "Nothing I use seems to work and I have spent hundreds of dollars on various products. It's really been frustrating. I have to be so careful what I use on my face."

I tried to be as tactful as I could. "Are you sure you have sensitive skin?" I asked.

"Well," she paused, "I always seem to have a reaction to products."

"What happens?" I continued.

"My skin gets red and rough and it loses its shine."

"How long has this been going on?"

"For several years. I noticed it shortly after I turned forty and I just thought it was the curse of being middle-aged. That's when we moved to Colorado. Oh, and I also had a hysterectomy the year after we moved."

I think she would have continued to talk about her surgically induced menopause but I decided to interject.

"Maybe you have dry skin and not sensitive skin. Maybe your skin changed after your surgery and your move."

"Do you think so? What does that mean for my skin?"

"If your skin is dry, not sensitive, it would mean that you need to focus on hydration and use products that can help your skin hold adequate moisture." I told her that it's important to balance her skin's sluggish oil production, along with supporting healthy collagen production. Enhancing the exfoliating process was also something to focus on, and I recommended that she use a gentle enzyme-based exfoliator that could actually stimulate collagen production for a more balanced, healthy glow. I told her that not only will regular exfoliation assist in collagen production it will also allow her nourishing creams to enter the skin with greater ease.

"Visualize a dry sponge and a moist sponge," I told her. "Which one will pick up the spills more readily?"

She immediately said, "The moist one."

"You want your skin to be like that moist sponge, picking up the nutrients from your nourishing cream," I explained.

The questions and metaphors continued and the flight flew by. Soon, we were landing in Colorado and she was relieved that she had finally figured out the truth about her skin type.

6

Effective Acne Treatment

Most people are surprised when I tell them that more than 60 million people are affected by acne. After talking with many people about their skin over the years, I am not surprised at all; however, there was a time that I would have been shocked.

As a teenager and young adult, I suffered with acne. Every morning my acne stared back at me as I looked in the mirror. It was not only physically disfiguring, but also emotionally depressing. I would never have believed there were 60 million other people just like me. When you have moderate to severe acne, you feel as if you are the only one in the world with pimples. I felt alone and isolated, branded with bad skin that everyone noticed. It was the first thing I saw in the morning and the last thought I had at night. I felt helpless and ugly, and always shied away from the camera.

But I am persistent. I was determined to heal my acne and I did not stop until my skin was clear. Since that time, I have perfected my acne treatment plan and I have seen it work on thousands of people over the years. I hope it can help you, too.

DEFINING ACNE

Acne is considered a subcategory of the oily skin type. It is the most common skin illness in the United States. According to the American Dermatologist Association, of the 60 million Americans who have acne, nearly 85 percent are aged twelve to twenty-four. However, adults get acne, too. It has been estimated that about 20 percent of the adult population has active acne.

Acne comes in many forms, including black- and whiteheads, severe nodules, or cysts. A small red inflammatory bump on the skin is known as a papule. A pustule is another name for a whitehead because of the pus formation. Acne is severe enough to cause scarring for more than 20 million Americans.

Acne is caused by one or more factors, including excess oil production, poor exfoliation, genetics, diet, stress, and hormones. Products we use on our face, especially oil-based cosmetics, can also cause acne.

Although excess oil production can cause acne, oil is actually good for the skin. Oils that are produced by the sebaceous glands in the skin help with lubrication and prevent water loss. In addition to the face, there are a number of sebaceous glands on the back, chest, and shoulders, which is why some people may develop acne in those areas. Poor cellular turnover, combined with excess oil production in these areas, causes clogging of skin pores, leading to acne. Dry brushing and using a loofah in the shower can help tremendously with dead skin cell exfoliation.

I'm often asked why acne is worse during puberty, menstruation, pregnancy, or perimenopause (the time leading up to menopause). All those

Categorizing Your Acne

Mild: Small spots that consist of blackheads and whiteheads and some pustules that are at or near the surface

Moderate: Numerous blackheads and whiteheads, as well as papules and pustules, covering from one-quarter to three-quarters of the face

Severe: Deep cysts, inflammation, extensive skin damage, and scarring

Note: A blackhead is when the pore is clogged and open, whereas a whitehead is when the pore is clogged and closed. Papules are small raised bumps, whereas pustules contain pus and can be any size.

times share a common component—increased hormone activity. Hormones directly affect oil production in the skin. The hormone fluctuations that occur in perimenopause and menopause can cause spikes in oil production. Similarly, increased hormone production during puberty, menstruation, and pregnancy can cause excess oil to be produced. When the skin has too much oil, the *propionium bacteria* (*P bacteria*) can flourish on the skin's surface, which can lead to acne if skin is not cleansed and exfoliated morning and evening. Infectious, painful acne is often a blend of trapped dead skin cells and dirt, increased oil production, and bacteria.

Acne is a treatable skin condition, but it takes time, patience, and persistence.

The combination of dead skin, dirt, and excessive oil creates fertile ground for the *P bacteria* to thrive and are at the heart of most acne problems. Over the years, I have found that normalizing oil production, promoting consistent cellular turnover (through exfoliation), and neutralizing the *P bacteria* alleviate most forms of acne. There are many nontoxic extracts and essential oils we can use on our skin that have amazing antioxidant and anti-inflammatory properties and can help heal acne as well.

Acne is a treatable skin condition, but it takes time, patience, and persistence. Acne can be controlled and even eliminated completely by following a comprehensive, natural treatment plan. Unfortunately, many people trying to control their acne resort to harsh prescription or over-the-counter medications that dry the skin and cause excess oil production, creating a vicious cycle. These medications can also lead to severely sensitive skin, premature aging, and permanent skin damage. Let's take a closer look at some of the most common ways conventional medicine treats acne.

CONVENTIONAL TREATMENT

Acne is typically treated with over-the-counter or prescription topical agents. In some severe cases, doctors may prescribe drugs, cortisone injections, and surgical removal (known as excision).

There are numerous over-the-counter acne products presently available. With 60 million people affected by this skin condition, acne is big business. Most of these medications contain one of the following active ingredients or ingredient combinations:

🐾 **benzoyl peroxide:** This ingredient is so drying that it has been shown to bleach hair, sheets, towels, and clothing, and it is recommended that you wear an old shirt when applying products with this ingredient. If this ingredient can do so much damage to your clothing, just imagine what it's doing to your skin!

🐾 **rescorcinol and sulfur:** Sulfur is often combined with other ingredients, even though we don't know exactly how it works. Rescorcinol should not be combined with anti-acne ingredients (other than sulfur), and can cause skin irritation.

🐾 **acetone:** This ingredient is incorporated in many anti-acne products. It is common knowledge that acetone is a cleaning agent and preservative, often used in nail polish remover and gasoline. I'm not sure why anyone would consider putting it on the skin.

🐾 **isopropyl alcohol:** Used in high concentrations, alcohol is too drying and sends the skin into a dry/oily roller coaster when used daily. Note that ethyl alcohol, used in minute quantities with balancing ingredients, can be effective in the right formula.

What's most distressing about these topical treatments is that they can make acne worse. They only focus on temporary symptom relief, rather than addressing the underlying causes. In the long run, they create an unhealthy cycle for the skin that includes episodes of severe dryness followed by periods of extreme oiliness.

An effective acne treatment program must accomplish three things:

1. gently exfoliate
2. normalize oil production
3. neutralize *P bacteria*

Over-the-counter topical treatments do not accomplish all three of these goals. When acne is severe, a dermatologist may prescribe a topical medication. Topical prescription medications may include:

- **benzoyl peroxide:** in a stronger, prescription form than the over-the-counter version

- **antibiotics:** to help slow the growth of bacteria

- **vitamin A derivatives (also known as retinoids):** an altered form of vitamin A, which may include tretinoin (Retin-A2), adapalene (Differin), and tazarotene (Tazorac)

- **sulfur-containing products:** it is believed that sulfur can help break down black- and whiteheads

These drugs can cause a variety of side effects, including stinging, burning, redness, scaling, peeling, and even skin discoloration. The most serious side effects come with the oral prescription drug isotretinoin (Accutane). According to the American Academy of Dermatology (AAD), "There have been a number of reported suicides and suicide attempts in people taking isotretinoin." This is especially troubling because this drug is often prescribed to teenagers, an age group with relatively high rates of depression and suicide already.

The AAD also reports that the following side effects can occur in people taking isotretinoin:

DID YOU KNOW?

There are more than 150 different types of antibiotic drugs now on the market. The use of antibiotics for acne is common. According to www.MayoClinic.com, "Antibiotics are the first line of defense against many infections. But overusing or misusing antibiotics can cause more harm than good, including antibiotic resistance." If you have to use an antibiotic, be sure to use it completely and follow it with a probiotic (acidophilus) supplement between meals for at least two weeks after you are done taking your antibiotic.

🦁 dry eyes, mouth, lips, nose, or skin (very common)

🦁 itching

🦁 nosebleeds

🦁 muscle aches

🦁 sun sensitivity

🦁 poor night vision

🦁 changes in the blood, such as higher cholesterol

🦁 change in liver function

I'm often asked about the safety of over-the-counter and prescription medications for acne. In some severe cases, these drugs or excision may be necessary; however, I have found that most of the time people with acne can alleviate their acne by means of a more comprehensive, nontoxic plan. In severe cases, I recommend microdermabrasion therapy before trying prescription medications. (For more information on microdermabrasion and laser therapy, see the inset on page 91.)

To get rid of acne, we need to look at the underlying cause and do more than address the pimples or blackheads on the surface. Let's contrast conventional treatment with a nontoxic, inside-out approach.

FROM THE OUTSIDE

Acne is an external condition. That's why most people want to deal with it from the outside first. From a topical perspective, begin with products that contain nontoxic ingredients. My effective anti-acne plan calls for a four-step strategy that includes using:

1. a nontoxic exfoliating cleanser with antibacterial ingredients and essential oils

2. a balancing toner with anti-inflammatory ingredients, such as hemamelis and turmeric

Microdermabrasion and Laser Treatments

The many side effects of prescription acne drugs, including antibiotic resistance, are prompting patients and doctors alike to look for alternative treatments—especially in cases of severe acne. As a result, medical procedures have been developed to treat acne.

Typically designed to reduce the signs of aging, both microdermabrasion and laser treatments are used with some success on individuals with moderate to severe acne. Although these treatments do not require a dermatologist, I recommend that they be performed by a medical esthetician. According to the American Society of Plastic Surgeons, microdermabrasion is a procedure in which a skin care professional "uses a devise like a fine sandblaster to spray tiny crystals across the face, mixing gentle abrasion with suction to remove the dead, outer layer of the skin." Skin can get tight and red following the treatment; however, the mild side effects do not last long. Microdermabrasion can help with acne because it deeply exfoliates as it opens trapped pores and removes oil and dirt deposits. It also enhances circulation of the skin. A number of studies have confirmed that many people with acne experience some improvement with microdermabrasion.

There are several types of laser resurfacing procedures as well. These techniques are similar to microdermabrasian; however, they are much more aggressive. Like microdermabrasion, laser resurfacing helps remove unwanted tissue on the skin's surface. Rather than using an abrasion technique, a polarized light is beamed via a laser. Laser resurfacing is expensive, and there are no federal restrictions as to who can perform it. If you opt for laser treatments, be sure to have it done only by an experienced medical esthetician or a licensed plastic surgeon or dermatologist.

3. a natural mud mask or exfoliating fruit pulp peel, such as a pumpkin peel, rich in natural, healing retinoids

4. a flavonoid-rich, hydrating renewal cream with essential oils, especially lemongrass and grapefruit, to calm and balance overactive oil glands

Following is a closer look at each of these steps, beginning with the most important step of all—cleansing. An effective acne treatment plan must include the use of a quality, nontoxic cleanser that can provide therapeutic benefits. The cleanser must not only exfoliate properly, it must have ingredients that can fight bacteria living on the skin's surface. There are many natural, nontoxic ingredients that have powerful antibacterial properties. Most notable is totarol extract from the totara tree in New Zealand. Tea tree oil is also an effective antibacterial agent, yet the antibacterial effects of totarol have been shown to be a thousand times more effective than those of tea tree oil. Salicylic acid, from pumpkin seeds and cranberry extract, also has powerful antibacterial effects. The ancient herb horopito, which comes from Australia, is also one of my favorite ingredients to neutralize the *P bacteria*. Horopito also has powerful antioxidant properties.

A cleanser specifically designed for oily skin should also contain essential oils to help reduce and normalize oil production. Essential oil of lemongrass is especially beneficial for oily skin and will help calm down overactive oil glands. Grapefruit essential oil also has some antibacterial effects. These essential oils also provide aromatherapy benefits. Cranberry extract is also recommended for its astringent and antioxidant properties. Acids, such as salicylic from pumpkin seeds and glycolic from rhubarb, are fantastic for ensuring normal cellular turnover and deep cleansing of the pores. Many of these essential oils are now available organically, meaning they are grown without the use of toxic pesticides and fertilizers.

Following a thorough exfoliating cleanse, the person with acne will benefit from a serum containing concentrated amounts of healing ingredients. The serum should contain totarol, salicylic acid, natural retinol, cranberry, tea tree oil, and other natural ingredients to help reduce blackheads, pore size, and cystic acne. Vitamin C serum can also be beneficial (be sure it contains a minimum of 10 percent stabilized L-ascorbic acid) to aid the skin in healing and reducing inflammation, therefore reducing scar tissue.

Superconcentrated fruit peels are great. Pumpkin, cranberry, apple, blueberry, and pineapple purées gently loosen and dissolve dead skin cells, stimulate collagen, and nourish the skin. A high-quality, nontoxic fruit concentrate peel will contain a variety of ingredients to support the activity of the enzymes in the fruits. This can include D-beta fructan, L-sodium hyaluronate, and L-malic acid. For more information about these ingredients, see Appendix B "Nourishing Ingredients," at the back of the book.

Overdrying the skin will pull debris into the pores (creating blackheads and whiteheads) and further into the skin, making it more difficult for the extraction or natural excretion of those impurities.

Mud masks containing bentonite and kaolin are also part of my acne treatment plan. Quality mud masks detoxify and provide healing minerals to the skin. Make sure the mud mask also contains rosemary essential oil and totarol. The mask should never completely dry the skin because that will cause dehydration.

An oil-free nourishing cream should be used in the morning and evening. It's not surprising that grapefruit, cranberry, and lemongrass provide the perfect backdrop for an effective anti-acne cream. Keep in mind that there is a big difference between oils we should avoid and natural essential oils. Essential oils are known as volatile oils because they dissipate so quickly. Some essential oils even have a balancing effect, meaning that when your skin is producing too much oil, oil production will be reduced and when your skin is not producing enough there are essential oils that will increase oil production. If a product states that it is OIL-FREE FOR OILY/ACNE SKIN, be sure it contains important natural essential oil extracts such as lavender, lemongrass, grapefruit, rosemary, clary, or juniper. B-vitamins (specifically pyridoxine, niacinamide, D-panthenol, and D-biotin) are also healing to skin with acne.

It's critical to use products that contain nontoxic ingredients so as not to add irritants to already compromised and irritated skin. Products that excessively strip the skin of its natural moisture can actually worsen acne. When the skin becomes dehydrated, it pulls the debris in the clogged pores deeper into the skin, making it almost impossible for easy extraction or natural discharge. Synthetic chemicals and toxic ingredients in skin care products can also increase inflammation and damage skin tissue. This adds insult to injury for already damaged, acne-ridden skin. Balancing the skin is not just important for oily/acne-prone skin, all skin types can benefit from properly formulated skin care products that focus on balanced oil production.

In addition to the four-step plan, here are some additional tips to follow that may help alleviate your acne:

- Don't squeeze pimples because that will just aggravate the inflammatory process and worsen acne.

- Be sure your pillowcase is washed in chemical-free detergents on a regular basis.

- Avoid using cosmetics that are petroleum-based and occlusive (clogging); they suffocate the skin and inhibit proper tissue respiration. When choosing color cosmetics, choose cosmetics that allow your skin to breathe. Mineral-based cosmetics are what I use and recommend. Make sure they do not contain artificial colors or synthetic fragrances.

- Avoid tanning booths, sunlamps, and excess sun exposure; tanning simply masks acne and can actually make it worse because of the added inflammation.

In order to heal acne, you must find ways to reduce inflammation from both the outside and inside. To give yourself the best chance of success, it is important to combine anti-inflammatory products with an anti-inflammatory diet.

FROM THE INSIDE

Treating acne from the inside, through diet and lifestyle, is crucial to achieving long-term, sustainable success. When it comes to diet, there are several aspects to consider, beginning with dairy and sugar. I used to think it was okay to eat as much bread as my stomach could hold. I didn't realize that the unused carbohydrates turned into sugar, which triggered production and secretion of insulin. This caused all sorts of problems, including problems with my skin.

All simple sugars, particularly in the form of soda, have been shown to contribute to acne. Author and clinician Ray Sahelian, MD, reminds his patients that, in addition to sugar, there are a variety of foods that will likely promote acne, including white breads, chips, processed foods made with flour, fried foods, and foods that contain trans- or hydrogenated fats. Fast foods should be avoided because of their high fat content.

Milk, milk products, margarine, shortening, and other synthetically hydrogenated vegetable oils are acne instigators as well. "Milk should be avoided not only because it contains transfatty acids, but also because it may contain trace levels of hormones," explains Michael Murray, ND, author of *Natural Alternatives to Over-the-Counter and Prescription Drugs*. If you choose to drink milk, I recommend only buying milk from organic, non–genetically modified sources. The label should state ORGANIC and/or NON-GMO, which stands for genetically-modified organism.

Many studies have found a positive association between milk intake and the developing or worsening of acne. Researchers from the Harvard School of Public Health concluded in the *Journal of the American Academy of Dermatology* that "The association with milk may be because of the pres-

Foods That Can Irritate Acne

- Dairy products (especially milk)
- Simple sugars (soda pop, candy, and other sweets)
- Refined carbohydrates (white bread, cereals, and other processed foods made with flour)
- Trans fats (French fries, chips)
- Chocolate (due to the high fat and sugar content in most brands)
- Nuts

ence of hormones and bioactive molecules in milk." Don't forget: Many dairy products, like cheese, sour cream, and cottage cheese, contain milk, so be sure those products are organic, too.

The acne connection is still another reason to drink hormone-free, organic milk whenever possible. Keep in mind, however, that individuals who have dairy allergies, should avoid drinking milk entirely, even organic milk. For those who are allergic to cow's milk, organic rice milk or almond milk are great alternatives.

Chocolate can also be problematic for those who struggle with acne because it is high in both sugar and fat. If you want to splurge, however, try dark chocolate with at least 50 percent cocoa. These chocolates are higher quality and also contain antioxidants. And if you are a chocolate lover, they taste great!

Food allergies can contribute to acne as well. In addition to chocolate and dairy, allergies to refined carbohydrates and nuts can worsen acne.

Iodized salt should also be avoided. "Foods high in iodized salt should be eliminated, as some people are quite sensitive to the iodine, a known cause of acne," according to Dr. Murray. "A healthful diet rich in natural whole foods like vegetables, fruits, whole grains, and beans is the first recommendation for treating acne."

I agree with Dr. Murray. A diet rich in organic vegetables and fruit, fresh wild fish, and fiber—and low in fat—is a great diet for someone who struggles with acne. In addition, drink plenty of purified water because it plays a very important role in detoxification and hydration. A minimum of eight, 8-ounce glasses of fresh, purified water daily is recommended. For more dietary advice, see the diet and lifestyle information in Chapter 9.

Dietary supplements incorporating anti-acne nutrients help complement a healthful diet. In his book *Natural Alternatives to Over-the-Counter and Prescription Drugs*, Dr. Murray recommends:

🦁 zinc: 30 to 45 mg daily

🦁 chromium: 200 mcg

🦁 selenium: 200 mcg daily

🦁 vitamin E: 200 to 400 IU daily

For women with premenstrual aggravation of acne, Dr. Murray recommends vitamin B_6, at a dose of 50 mg, three times a day. Vitamin A has been shown to alleviate acne. Because of the high doses of vitamin A required and the potential toxicity of those dosages (100,000 to 400,000 IU daily), it should not be used without supervision from a medical professional. A safe dosage of vitamin A is 25,000 IU daily. Vitamin A works synergistically with zinc and vitamin E.

Remember, dietary supplements are just that—supplements to the diet. For clear skin, start with a healthful diet and build from there.

ACNE TREATMENT THAT WORKS

I know firsthand the pain and embarrassment that can come from having acne. Acne can be emotionally, as well as physically, devastating. Through dietary changes and the use of nontoxic skin care products, most people I have worked with are able to completely alleviate their acne, and not only reclaim their beautiful vibrant skin, but also their self-esteem. Clear skin is possible using a nontoxic, comprehensive approach.

Sun exposure is the next challenge that needs to be addressed. The following chapter will take a much closer look at how the sun affects our skin.

Along the Journey

Acute Acne for Fifteen Years

I have received a lot of letters over the years. Many of them are from people who have struggled with acne. Some of the stories are heartbreaking. So many people have been scarred by acne, not just physically but emotionally. They explain that their acne has affected their self-confidence and that they don't feel comfortable socially or professionally. They are desperate to get some relief from their acne.

While all the letters are special, one in particular stands out. It was from a thirty-five-year-old woman who had had acne on and off since she was in her teens. I could relate to her frustration. In her letter she said that, without fail, every time she had some big event planned, she would have a breakout. In between breakouts, she said her skin was red, dry, and painful. She said that even when her skin was clear, she was miserable because of the harsh side effects of the prescription medication she was using. The skin on her face became so red and sensitive that she resorted to using petroleum jelly just to get a little relief from the stinging. She was afraid that her skin would be permanently damaged. And then she got pregnant.

She actually had to stop using the prescription drug when she got pregnant because of its toxicity. From that point on, she was determined to find some other way to control her acne and heal her sensitive skin.

As she worked on losing weight after her baby was born, she became more diligent about her diet. She found a way to rid herself of cravings for sweets, and she reduced the amount of refined carbohydrates she ate. She was very careful about the products she used on her child, which carried over to all the products she used, including her own skin care products. She changed her skin care routine dramatically and began using a nontoxic cleanser and nourishing cream twice a day. She used a fruit peel three times a week and was also fairly consistent about applying a healing serum after she cleansed and before she put on her nourishing cream.

At the time of her letter, her son was two years old and she was happy to report that her acne was gone completely and her skin continues to heal from the damage the drug caused. It was obvious after reading her letter that she was very proud of her effort. "I made this a priority in my life and I am no longer tortured by my horrible bouts of acne," she wrote. Her persistence is inspiring. Sometimes it's not easy getting rid of acne, but it is possible.

7 *Sun Care*

The sun fascinates me. Sunshine is vital to life and yet its power can do so much damage. Although most of us like to spend time outdoors, the sun is your skin's worst enemy. Sun exposure is the primary cause of premature aging, brown spots, wrinkles, and skin cancer.

If you are a trivia buff, here are some interesting facts about the sun you can share at your next dinner party.

- The sun is located 93 million miles from the earth.

- If you could drive to the sun from the earth at sixty miles per hour (97 kmph), it would take you 176 years to get there.

- It takes more than eight minutes for sunlight to actually reach the earth once it leaves the sun.

The sun is so far away and yet some days it appears as if it's right on top of us. With such an expanse between the earth and the sun, how can it do so much damage? The power of the sun should never be underestimated. The sun itself is sixteen times hotter than boiling water. But it's not just the heat: It's what else the sun emits that can do the most damage—ultraviolet (UV) radiation. There is no question that ultraviolet radiation from the sun is dangerous. The ozone layer near the Earth's surface can deflect ultraviolet radiation; however, it cannot absorb all the radiation emitted by the sun. In addition, pollution (greenhouse gases) continues to deplete

DID YOU KNOW?

Compared to the Earth, the sun is huge. For perspective, if the sun were the size of a basketball, the Earth would be the size of the head of a pin! The sun is the largest, most powerful object in our solar system.

the ozone layer, exposing us to more ultraviolet radiation than ever before.

There are three types of ultraviolet radiation—UVA, UVB, and UVC—depending on the wavelength. About 99 percent of the radiation that reaches the earth is UVA. While UVA rays do not produce sunburn, as UVB rays do, this form of radiation still contributes to aging skin and skin cancer. UVB rays, while in limited quantity, are more intense and cause sunburn.

DAMAGING EFFECTS

At some point, all of us have had a tan or felt the pain and sting of sunburn. A suntan is actually the skin's response to sun exposure. It's the skin's way of trying to create a canopy of shade to protect vulnerable live skin cells. Melanin is produced by melanocytes and secreted through dendrites (tentacle-like structures on the end of the cell) then deposited on top of our healthy cells like tiny hats to protect them, much like the protection you get from wearing a hat on your head. Sunburn is an inflammatory condition created when the sun's ultraviolet rays penetrate the skin's inner layer, breaking down the skin's key support structures—collagen and elastin. Just as the term implies, the sun actually *burns* our delicate skin tissue.

In reality, there is no such thing as a "healthy tan." The pink or red color of sunburn is actually inflamed, damaged skin. Getting sunburned, however, is not the only indication of skin damage. Even people with a tan experience skin damage from the sun. Repeated insults to the skin, such as sunburns or deep tans, can cause scar tissue and loss of elasticity. Ultimately, skin will become thick, unable to retain water, and void of collagen and elastin. That's what causes skin to look like leather.

Hyperpigmentation, also known as age spots, and melasma are side effects of repeated, unprotected sun exposure. Melasma is a skin condition characterized by patches of tan or dark spots on the face. It is most common in women who are pregnant, taking oral contraceptives, or undergoing hormone replacement therapy. Women who are experiencing these types of hormonal fluctuations may be more sensitive to sun exposure, and develop melasma as a result. Genetic predisposition can also play a role in melasma. If you have a family history of hyperpigmention or melasma, you should be especially diligent about protecting your skin from the sun.

It has been estimated that sun exposure causes up to 90 percent of the visible signs of aging skin, including wrinkles, age spots, and broken capillaries. This makes sense because the sun can directly damage collagen and elastin, the two most important youth-enhancing structures of the skin. Excessive sun exposure is also dehydrating, which contributes to older-looking, photodamaged skin (*photo* in this context, refers to the sun).

Photoaging and *photodamage* are really the same thing. They both refer to changes in the appearance and function of the skin, caused by repeated exposure to the sun rather than merely the passage of time. I'll discuss photodamage and aging in more detail in the next chapter.

Sun Care Facts

- Snow, sand, water, concrete, and glass can all reflect sunlight.
- Clouds do not protect you from damaging ultraviolet rays.
- The higher the altitude, the more intense the sun gets (about 6 percent for every 1,000 feet).
- The sun's ultraviolet rays can penetrate many types of clothing, but you can now purchase clothing with an SPF rating (for more information on this, visit www.sunprecautions.com).
- Dry, dehydrated skin burns more easily than well-hydrated skin.
- The sun can damage your eyes, increasing your risk of cataracts, macular degeneration, and eyelid cancers (see inset on page 105).

There is no question that the most troubling and dangerous effect of sun exposure is skin cancer.

SKIN CANCER

"Collectively, skin cancers are the most common forms of cancer," explain the authors of the *Definitive Guide to Cancer*. "More than 1 million cases of nonmelanoma skin cancers are diagnosed each year; about 800,000 are basal-cell carcinoma, a tumor of the epidermis, usually with a molelike appearance, that is seldom metastatic (having spread); the remainder are squamous-cell skin cancer, tumors originating from the most superficial layer of the epithelium."

There are a variety of symptoms of skin cancer, including changes in skin pigmentation, new or changing skin growths, or changes in moles. Skin cancers can be tender, itchy, scaly, and can even have some discharge. A biopsy (a tissue sample examined by a pathologist under a microscope) is the only way to confirm skin cancer.

> **DID YOU KNOW?**
>
> *More than 1 million people in the United States are diagnosed with some form of skin cancer each year.*

"The single greatest risk factor for all forms of skin cancer is exposure to ultraviolet radiation from the sun," notes the *Definitive Guide to Cancer*. "Protecting the skin with sunblock, clothing, a hat, and shade is the best way to prevent skin cancer and help ensure it doesn't reoccur."

The authors of the *Definitive Guide to Cancer* also suggest a diet high in antioxidants, such as vitamins A, C, E, and beta-carotene, as a way to avoid skin cancer. Using antioxidants topically can also help when it comes to preventing skin cancer. According to a report in the *Journal of the American Academy of Dermatology*, there are several nutrients that have been identified as anti–skin cancer agents, both orally and topically, including EGCG (from green tea), grape seed extract, curcumin (from turmeric), lycopene (found in tomatoes), and the trace mineral selenium.

I'm often asked about the safety of tanning beds. Many people are under the mistaken impression that tanning beds are safe alternatives to sun exposure. While tanning beds are designed to emit fewer UVB rays—the rays that cause sunburn—they still emit UVA rays. The argument is that, because UVA rays don't burn the skin, they cause no damage. There is clear evidence, however, that UVA rays increase the risk of skin cancer, particularly the more dangerous form of skin cancer known as melanoma. UVA rays are also a strong immune suppressant, allowing skin cancers to spread more rapidly.

I firmly believe that unprotected, excessive sun exposure over the years —combined with the proliferation of environmental and cosmetic toxins— is to blame for the significant increase of skin cancers. The diagnosis of skin cancer is happening at a younger age. Some believe that toxins in sunscreens used on children may be contributing to childhood skin cancers.

In 2000, the National Toxicity Program and the National Institutes of Health added tanning beds and sunlamps to the list of known cancer-causing agents. Many studies have confirmed the link between skin cancer and "intentional exposure to ultraviolet radiation" (through tanning beds and sunbathing).

The takeaway message on tanning beds and sunbathing is this: No, they are not safe. Instead, I highly recommend, the "fake" tan. Self-tanning products are the fastest-growing segment of the sun care market, report the authors of *Sun Protection for Life*. Having a sun-soaked, tan exterior is way overrated. But if you are looking for that fashionable tan, try a high-quality, self-tanning product that does not contain toxic ingredients. I just started using a self-tanner and I love the way it makes me look. I also love the fact that I can look tan without being exposed to damaging UV rays.

Keep in mind that the only approved self-tanning active ingredient is dihydroxyacetone (DHA), from sugar beets. Erythrulose from red raspberries works synergistically with DHA to extend the life of the sunless tan. A quality sunless tanning product should also contain essential oils and ingredients to hydrate, moisten, and soften the skin, including safflower, aloe, grapefruit, orange, and allantoin from comfrey.

If you are using a self-tanning product, you still have to use sunblock. Products that give you a fake tan, do not provide sun protection.

PROTECTION

When it comes to sun exposure the bottom line is this: Protect yourself or pay the price. Proper protection begins with the appropriate topical product.

Many people are confused about the difference between a sunblock and a sunscreen. A sunblock lies on the surface of the skin and provides a physical shield that reflects the sun's UV rays. A sunscreen, on the other hand, penetrates the skin and, when activated (about fifteen to twenty minutes after the application), absorbs ultraviolet rays for a limited time. The higher the SPF (sun protection factor) number on a sunscreen, the more chemicals it contains. I recommend sunblocks, rather than sunscreens, because they work as long as they are on the skin. Sunscreens, on the other hand, become neutralized quickly and, depending on the SPF rating, need to be reapplied often. I am also uncomfortable with many of the toxic ingredients in sunscreens, which are being absorbed by the skin. Whether you use sunscreen or sunblock, it's important for the product to provide both UVA and UVB protection. To avoid toxic chemicals found in most sunscreens, I recommend a mineral-based sunblock.

The most significant factor associated with sunscreens or sunblocks is their sun protection factor. SPF is not a direct indication of how much more time you can spend in the sun. SPF is defined as the amount of time it would take your skin to redden with sun protection as opposed to without. For example, if a product has an SPF of 30, it will take your skin thirty times longer to redden by using the product than it would without the product. If your skin would typically get red within ten minutes without sunscreen, it will stay protected for up to five hours (30 x 10 = 300 minutes ÷ 60 = 5 hours) with the SPF 30 sunblock.

It is important to wear a sunblock even on cloudy days. "Though not as bright as sunny days, much of the harmful UV light still comes through [on cloudy days]," according to the University Corporation for Atmospheric Research, which also reports that "having a tan is little protection from skin damage, providing an SPF of only about 2."

Although products with a higher SPF provide you with longer protection, you should reapply sunscreen or sunblock frequently if you are sweating or in and out of water. This is especially true if you are using a sunscreen as opposed to a sunblock. Remember, a sunscreen's ingredients need time to become activated, and then they only last for a limited time. The action of a sunblock is different, however, because it contains zinc oxide and sits on the top of the skin, shielding skin cells from harmful UV rays.

If the sunblock you are using is free of toxic ingredients and contains natural therapeutic agents, it will help preserve the skin's moisture without clogging pores or irritating eyes. Effective sunblock ingredients are zinc oxide and titanium dioxide (0.67 percent). A sunblock that contains micronized zinc oxide at 11.6 percent will not leave your skin looking ghostly white, as many zinc oxide products will.

Protecting Your Eyes and Lips

In addition to your skin, you need to protect your lips and eyes from the sun. According to the University Corporation for Atmospheric Research, "People who don't protect their eyes when they are young run the risk of loss of sight when older, including getting cataracts." Sun exposure to the eyes can also cause melanoma (cancer) of the eye, as well as increase your risk of macular degeneration, a disease that can destroy the retina. To protect your eyes, it is important to consistently wear sunglasses that filter 100 percent of the ultraviolet light, especially during midday peak sun times. Infants and children should also wear eye protection. It may be difficult to get them to keep sunglasses on, but your patience and persistence will be worth it.

Don't forget to protect your lips. Use a lip treatment that blocks the UVA and UVB rays from the sun. Lip balm will help protect against burning, chapping, drying, and lip cancer. I recommend a nontoxic lip treatment that contains titanium dioxide to block the sun, as well as antioxidants, Melissa extract, and nourishing shea and kokum butters.

Some other natural ingredients to look for in a nontoxic sunblock include:

🜚 caprylic acid from coconut oil because it has good spreading properties

🜚 D-alpha tocopherol (natural vitamin E), a powerful skin antioxidant

🜚 aloe extract for hydration, softening, and anti-inflammatory actions

🜚 allantoin from comfrey, which is soothing and healing to the skin

🜚 squalane from olives to prevent skin dehydration

To apply your mineral sunblock, place a dollop of the product in the palm of your hand, rub your hands together vigorously, and gently press the sunblock on your face and all exposed skin.

The book *Sun Protection for Life* reports that most individuals underapply their sunblock by as much as 50 percent. Don't be afraid to apply sun protection products liberally. After all, if you don't use the product, it definitely won't work! Remember to always protect children. The sunburns that occur at a young age are the most dangerous and can lead to skin cancer in the years to come.

IT'S NEVER TOO LATE

The sun is a complex ball of fire that can provide outdoor enthusiasts with a lot of fun and enjoyment, but it can also be far more dangerous than you may realize. If you take proper precautions, you can safely enjoy the great outdoors and the sun.

Here are some important points to remember about sun exposure and protection:

1. Too much sun can accelerate aging and cause skin cancer.

2. Use nontoxic, safe, sunless tanning products as healthy alternatives to sunbathing and tanning booths.

3. The best way to protect your skin is with a quality, nontoxic sunblock that offers both UVA and UVB protection.

4. If you use a sunscreen, no matter what the SPF, you have to reapply it frequently.

5. Your sunblock is no different than your other body care products—it should contain healing, therapeutic ingredients that are nontoxic yet effective.

For more sun care tips, see the inset "Additional Sun Care Tips" below. A diligent sun care routine should be established as early in life as possible. The good news, however, is that it's never too late to start wearing a sunblock. Daily use of the right sun protection products can actually reverse a significant portion of sun damage. Take care of your skin by protecting it from the sun. You'll not only help prevent skin cancer, you'll keep your skin looking younger longer.

Additional Sun Care Tips

- Guard against sun damage in newborns and children by giving them extra protection from the sun.

- Remember to apply sunblock to your ears and the tops of your feet.

- Peak time for harmful UV radiation from the sun is between 10 a.m. and 4 p.m.

- Wear a wide-brimmed hat to protect your face, ears, and scalp; a baseball cap will only protect your forehead and nose!

- Wear sunglasses to protect your eyes.

- Use nontoxic, mineral-based sunblock.

- Use a self-tanner to achieve a tan.

- Do not use Retin-A, or even natural forms of vitamin A, if you are planning to spend time in the sun.

Along the Journey

Sun-Damaged Skier

Living in the Colorado Rockies, I have encountered many sun-damaged faces. While skiing one day, I met a woman who had the worst case of sun damage that I had ever seen. Her face looked like worn leather. We shared a lift together and started talking.

She asked me where I was from and I told her I had been living in Colorado for many years. She complimented me on my skin and said she never would have guessed I'd been living in a sunny state like Colorado so long because my skin didn't show it. I told her that I used to live in Arizona for many years. "I unknowingly abused my skin," I told her. "I've had to work really hard at reversing the hyperpigmentation and those premature fine lines." I didn't have to say anything about her skin because she brought it up.

"How old do you think I am?" she asked. I always get nervous when someone asks me this. Unfortunately, my guess was fifteen years higher than her actual age. I was mortified and apologetic.

She was very unhappy with the way her skin was aging. She loved the sun. "I think I'm addicted to being tan," she admitted. "What did you do to reverse the damage?"

She became my new ski buddy as we skied several runs together and I shared my skin secrets with her. I told her that the first thing she needed to do was wear a sunblock. I told her she could also use a self-tanner to get the tan she loved. She needed to exfoliate with a pumpkin peel to stimulate more collagen production and refine her skin's texture. I also told her to use a vitamin C serum that contained at least 10 percent L-ascorbic acid. A few weeks later, she called my office and thanked me for my advice. She said she was seeing improvements and she was even getting compliments from friends and family. She said I won't even recognize her the next time we share a chairlift together. I haven't seen her since, but I could tell in her voice that she felt more comfortable with how her skin looked and felt.

Age-Defying Skin Care

8

I have always been surprised by the popularity of the term *anti-aging*. It seems like an odd thing to promote. *Aging* means to change with time. Sure, we would all like to slow down the aging process or age gracefully with as much vitality as possible, but I'm not sure it is appropriate to say that we are "anti" aging. I prefer the term *healthy aging*.

If you search the term *anti-aging* on the Internet you will get millions of hits. As it turns out, to be "against" aging is big business. There are anti-aging academies, networks, guides, creams, supplements, procedures, books, and countless other ways to supposedly stop the aging process. Baby boomers throughout the world are desperate to live longer and look younger. Most of us want even more than that—we want to *feel* younger.

We have all seen people who have had undergone Botox treatment or plastic surgery: They have smoother skin but they don't necessarily look younger (for more information on Botox, see page 118). That's because they have merely ironed out their surface wrinkles; they haven't done anything to address the underlying issues of aging skin. The solution is not a quick fix; it's a comprehensive approach that supports and heals the infrastructure of the skin. Before we examine the solution, let's take a closer look at the problem.

THE PROBLEM

As discussed in previous chapters, our skin lives and breathes, just as we do. Skin cells have a short life expectancy but are constantly being replaced by new, healthy cells. This continual, dynamic process is what allows us to influence the health of our skin. In addition to maintaining the pace of skin cell turnover, our skin also battles the elements, such as sun, wind, and snow. Over time, our skin cells get tired. Remember, when we are younger, the average life span of a skin cell is about twenty-eight days. By the time we hit middle age, it's thirty-five days. When we move into retirement, the skin cell's life cycle grows even longer, which means we have many more "older" skin cells than ever before. That's why it's so important to support the skin as we age.

Aging is inherent to living. There is a built-in, internal system that automatically causes us to age. Short of death, there's nothing we can do to actually stop the aging process. In addition, there's a genetic component to aging. Some people are lucky to have inherited the healthy aging gene. But even they need to be aware of the factors that can influence skin aging. And for those who do not have that priceless gene on their family tree, there are many controllable variables that will help slow down the aging process and contribute to healthy aging.

In addition to decreased cell turnover and genetics, the automatic aging of the skin is due to a variety of complex factors, including (but not limited to):

- sun exposure
- inflammation
- oxygen depletion
- destruction of collagen and elastin
- reduced hormonal activity
- free radical damage
- fewer fat cells

Research demonstrates that key water-retaining and texture-enhancing compounds in the skin, such as hyaluronic acids and polysaccharides, become depleted as we age. Collagen and elastin, which give skin its firmness when we are young, become damaged, and we produce less of them as we age. Chronic inflammation, both internal and external, also damages skin and causes it to age more rapidly. Inflamed skin causes wrinkles and other skin aging issues.

The combination of these factors contributes to aging skin and can cause fine lines, wrinkles, changes in pigmentation such as age spots, also known as hyperpigmentation (dark spots or patches on the skin), and sagging skin. The skin also becomes thinner as we age, making it more susceptible to further damage. Thinner skin is more sensitive, dry, and looks more transparent; just the opposite of the plump, rosy, and glowing skin of our youth.

When it comes to the visible signs of aging, our face is like a billboard. Wrinkles and deepening expression lines on the face call out to everyone we interact with. As a society, we have come to abhor wrinkles. For some reason, most Americans value—and obsess over—a smooth complexion and youthful-looking skin. It's that obsession that has created the multi-billion-dollar anti-aging boom.

What actually causes wrinkles? Wrinkles form as the skin ages due to genetic predisposition, exposure to environmental elements—particularly the sun—and how we care for our skin. Here are some specific factors that can cause skin to wrinkle prematurely:

- smoking
- sun exposure and sun damage
- stress
- dehydration
- acne and some skin diseases
- facial muscle movement (frowning, smiling, etc.)
- loss of collagen and elastin due to early hysterectomy

In addition to fine lines and wrinkles, skin can also sag as it ages. This typically occurs around the eyes, the jaw line, and the neck. The upper lip can become thin as we age due to the loss of collagen, elastin, and fat cells under the skin.

The good news is that even as we age, we are still creating new, youthful skin cells. Doris Day, MD, author of *Forget the Facelift*, reminds us, "That's why, no matter how old you are and no matter how much damage has already been done to your skin, you can have younger-looking skin in a very short time." However, that's only possible if we have a healthy skin routine.

THE SOLUTION

If you can afford one product to prevent aging skin, it should be a sunblock. In the previous chapter we learned about the many dangers of sun exposure. The sun is the biggest culprit when it comes to the wrinkles and hyperpigmentation of aging skin. The only way to prevent this is to wear sunblock (for more information on sun protection, see Chapter 7).

In addition to using a sunblock, there are many healthy aging solutions to consider. These solutions fall into the following categories:

1. Topical treatments and skin care routines

2. Resurfacing

3. Cosmetic surgery and other medical treatments

I am a firm believer in the natural medicine motto: "First do no harm." That means that we should always try the least invasive, safest possible solution before jumping to dramatic surgeries and potentially toxic treatments. To first do no harm, we need to begin by considering topical treatments and adopting a healthy aging skin care routine. This will ensure that we are addressing the underlying causes of aging skin.

Healthy aging ingredients in topical treatments include:

🦋 retinoids

🦋 antioxidants such as vitamins A and C and resveratrol

🦎 alpha hydroxy and beta hydroxy acids

🦎 polypeptides such as AC-DermaPeptide MicroC from capsicum, AC-DermaPeptide Revitalizing from rice, Thymulen 4, Proteasyl TP, SYN-TACKS, SYN-COLL, and epidermal growth factor

🦎 plant extracts, including resveratrol from grapes, astaxanthin from the Hawaiian micro algae H. puvialis, cloudberry from the Arctic, and levisticum officionale from Persia, also called loveage

Choosing the Right Moisturizer

I prefer to think of moisturizers as nourishing creams. A well-formulated nourishing cream free of toxic ingredients should be the foundation of your skin care routine. Your nourishing cream needs to replenish the natural moisture in the outermost layer of the skin and protect the existing moisture content, while supporting the infrastructure of the skin. There are three key issues to focus on when choosing the right nourishing cream:

1. **Hydration.** Look for a product that contains squalane, cactus flower extract, cassia beta glycan, and L-sodium hyaluronate to hydrate the skin.

2. **Antioxidant activity.** Resveratrol, EGCG, retinol, and tocotrienols (vitamin E) are among the most potent healthy anti-aging antioxidant ingredients.

3. **Collagen production.** L-sodium hyaluronate, AC-DermaPeptide Micro C, SYN-COLL, Proteasyl TP, and Thymulen 4 all boost collagen production to help minimize fine lines and wrinkles.

Your nourishing cream should not be heavy, oily, or greasy. It should be thoroughly absorbed by the skin and leave a dewy, rose petal feel. It should also contain essential oils, such as rose, neroli, and bergamot, to enhance oil production.

Nature knows how to heal our skin. A variety of natural ingredients have direct healthy aging properties. For more information on specific ingredients and their benefits, see the chart on page 123.

The focus of the healthy aging skin care routine should be on rehydration and repair. As mentioned in previous chapters, keeping skin hydrated is critical no matter what your skin type or your age. It becomes even more important, however, as we age. The more mature the skin is, the dryer it will become. Lack of moisture not only leads to inflammation, which can damage skin, it is also a key cause of prematurely aging skin. Supple, soft skin requires proper hydration. In addition, as we age, our oil glands gradually produce less oil, naturally contributing to the skin's moisture loss.

Drinking plenty of fresh, purified water will help prevent dehydration. Using a natural, nontoxic, nourishing cream at least twice a day will help replenish natural moisture but also helps retain moisture that is already present in the skin. For more information on how to choose the most effective moisturizing and nourishing cream, refer to page 113. It's also important to consider your climate (see inset on page 115).

In addition to a nourishing cream, it's wise to use an all-natural hydrating mist throughout the day. The right mist should contain ingredients that help hydrate, nourish, and provide anti-inflammatory ingredients for the skin. An ingredient called heavy water (see page 59) is very important. Heavy water is from deep in the ocean and is a potent hydrating ingredient because it has a higher evaporation point than regular water. Other important mist ingredients include D-beta glucosamine from Chinese foxglove, fruit enzymes, turmeric, and antioxidants.

Using the proper skin care products can also help you directly repair the skin. Ingredients that help repair damaged skin include the peptides mentioned previously.

Over the years, I have been able to help many people protect their skin from accelerated aging or help them ease the symptoms associated with aging skin. Two key products that I recommend are a nourishing cream and a collagen-supporting serum. Most people take multivitamins and additional accessory vitamins to address their specific nutritional needs. A nourishing cream is like a multivitamin for the skin. Serums are akin to more specific and targeted accessory vitamins, such as CoQ_{10} and lutein. Serums are layered on the skin after cleansing.

Here is the healthy aging skin care routine that I recommend:

🦊 **Cleanse.** Use an exfoliating cleanser in the morning and evening.

🦊 **Apply serums.**

1. After cleansing in the morning and evening, use a vitamin C antioxidant combination serum (remember, it has to have at least 10 percent L-ascorbic acid). That can be combined with a hydrating serum with L-sodium hyaluronate or a firming serum containing L-proline and copper peptides.

Climate Changes Everything

Can the climate where you live cause wrinkles? According to a study conducted in Japan, even when the skin is exposed to low-humidity/dry climates for a short period, the skin loses its moisture content. Because lack of moisture contributes to wrinkles, the researchers concluded that exposure of human skin to a dry environment may contribute to an increase in skin wrinkling. It's crucial to consider your climate when developing your skin care routine.

The winter is an especially dry time of the year. According to a *Science Daily* report, the National Health Interview Survey (NHIS) reports that at least 81 million Americans experience dry, itchy, or scaly skin during the winter months. This is due to dryer, colder air and overheated homes and offices. "Keeping warm is a priority," says Rebecca A. Kazin, MD, assistant professor of dermatology and director of the Johns Hopkins Cosmetic Center. "But it sucks the moisture out of your skin."

Kazin's prescription is "moisture, moisture, moisture." She recommends using a humidifier and says, "Proper moisturizing is job one."

2. Also use a multipeptide serum that contains Thymulen 4, SYN-TACKS, SYN-COLL, Proteasyl TP, and essential growth factors.

- **Tone.** At various times throughout the day, spray a fruit enzyme mist on your face to tone the skin and keep it hydrated. This also acts as an anti-inflammatory and prepares the skin to receive nutrients from your nourishing cream.
- **Nourish.** Use a nourishing repair cream at least twice a day that contains antioxidants, such as resveratrol, astaxanthin, green tea (EGCG), peptides, and essential oils. Pay special attention to the skin around the eyes (for more information about eye creams, see the inset below).
- **Apply masks.** Twice a week use a hydrating mask that contains antioxidant berries, such as blueberries. For additional support you may want to use a detoxifying kaolin mud mask once a month.
- **Exfoliate.** Once a week use a gentle yet effective exfoliant, such as a pumpkin or a multifruit-based peel, that contains naturally occurring enzymes and acids.

The Eyes Have It!

The skin around the eyes is five to ten times thinner than skin on the rest of the face. There is also almost no oil production in this area. As we age, this skin can become even more problematic. Using a nontoxic eye cream twice a day will help hydrate and lubricate this sensitive tissue. Be sure the cream is nonocclusive, meaning it will allow the skin to breathe. Proper respiration is especially important for this tissue. Be sure the cream does not sting and will not cause blurry vision. Some eye creams seep into the eye socket and can cause problems, especially if you wear contact lenses. It's absolutely critical to avoid toxic ingredients (as listed in Chapter 2). Look for a cream that contains natural healing ingredients, such as liquid crystals from corn silk, aloe, and hyaluronic acid.

Age spots and random dark patches on the skin are issues that many individuals struggle with as they age. There are several all-natural ingredients that can help alleviate this issue, such as daisy, Applephenon™, gallic acid (abundantly present in the leaves of witch hazel, the flower of mango, pomegranate, and rhubarb), L-arbutin, L-lactic acid, L-ascorbic acid, and kojic acid.

When it comes to topical treatments and skin care routines, here are the most important things to remember:

1. Use products that contain nontoxic ingredients. Toxic chemicals, such as parabens, phthalates, urea, propylene glycol, and coloring agents, not only damage the skin, they can cause it to look older (for more information on toxic ingredients, see Chapter 2).

2. Consistency is important, so be sure to make healthy skin care a part of your daily routine.

3. Buy products from a manufacturer you trust, one that also has solid customer support.

4. Follow the dietary and lifestyle advice in the next chapter.

5. Be gentle on your skin. Use light pressure and try not to rub and pull on it when applying your products.

6. Use a mineral-based sunblock every day

The next chapter describes how your diet can help your skin look and feel younger. Some studies have even linked a poor diet to wrinkles on the face. Australian researchers found that individuals who ate more vegetables, olive oil, fish, and legumes had fewer wrinkles than those who ate butter, margarine, milk products, and sugar. It is believed that healthy, nutrient-rich foods help protect the skin and make it more resistant to the sun's harmful UV rays. Another study found that foods high in carotenoids, which are the compounds that give fruits and vegetables their color, also helped protect the skin from sun damage.

To fend off the early signs of aging skin, begin by using effective topical treatments and following a comprehensive skin care routine.

MEDICAL TREATMENTS

In some cases, topical treatments and changing your skin care routine may not be enough. Even if you choose to use a medial treatment, you still must focus on using safe and effective topical products while creating a healthy skin care routine.

To remove age spots, freckles, melasma, fine lines, and wrinkles, you can use one or more of the medical techniques presently available. The treatments that I endorse include alpha hydroxy and beta hydroxy acid chemical peels, dermabrasion or microdermabrasion, laser resurfacing, or intense pulsed light (IPL). Here is a description of each:

Botox is Bad Medicine

An article in the *New York Times* reported that there are about 1 million Americans using Botox. They spent an estimated $370 million on the injections in 2005. An MSN article estimated that $450 million was spent in 2007. What exactly are all these people injecting into their faces? Some have called it the most toxic bacteria ever discovered. It's botulinum toxin A, derived from bacterium botulinum—the same bacteria that causes botulism, a poisonous illness that can lead to paralysis and even death.

As it turns out, when injected into the skin, Botox paralyzes the muscles, evening out fine lines and wrinkles. It's no wonder people who use Botox look expressionless. Their faces are literally paralyzed. The treatment is temporary, prompting people to continually and addictively get more Botox injections. There are no studies that demonstrate the long-term safety of such a vicious cycle. Even if you can overlook the unknowns associated with long-term use of this toxin, there are direct dangers linked to having just one injection. As people flock to Botox clinics throughout the United States, unlicensed, unsafe concentrations of the product are making their way into the faces of unsuspecting con-

Chemical peels. This technique applies one or more chemicals to the face. The chemicals "burn" away damaged skin. This works especially well with photodamaged skin (prematurely aged skin as a result of sun exposure) and removing pigmentation discolorations. Chemical peels can help create a more even skin tone. Chemical peels also work on superficial and medium-depth fine lines and wrinkles. It can improve the skin's texture as it removes several layers of damaged skin cells. There is superficial skin injury following the procedure in the form of redness and swelling, similar to sunburn. Typically, the redness and swelling will go away in about forty-eight hours. More intense peels may cause symptoms of inflammation that can last up to a week. You can get peels more than once; however,

sumers. In 2006, four people nearly died after being injected with "black market" Botox at a dose nearly three thousand times the estimated human lethal dose. The scientific literature also contains reports of retinal tears and other eye injuries associated with Botox injections.

In addition, the Humane Society of the United States has filed several complaints against the FDA, seeking Botox testing information. The Humane Society states that every batch of Botox must be tested on animals, which causes "differing levels of muscular paralysis. Those [animals] given a high or powerful dose eventually die from suffocation, after their respiratory muscles become paralyzed." According to reports on Botox used in animal testing, these tests are barbaric. The animals are injected with Botox at varying dosages. The animals that have no paralysis did not get enough Botox and the animals that die received too much. The animals in the middle help determine the proper dosage. And that takes place every time a batch of Botox is whipped up!

Botox is a toxin that can be dangerous. What's worse is that production is associated with animal abuse. In my view, it should only be used when medically necessary—not as a temporary quick fix for facial lines and wrinkles.

What's the Difference between a Prune and a Plum?

Water! Would you rather look like a prune or a plum? I would rather look like a plum. So that means I want to use a nourishing cream that hydrates my skin. Collagen-boosting nutrients will also help the skin hold moisture and plump up those fine lines and wrinkles.

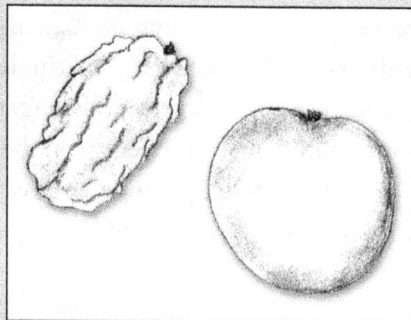

Which would you rather look like?

for moderate-depth peels, it is wise to wait three to six months between peels.

Dermabrasion and microdermabrasion. As we learned in the last chapter, these techniques can also be used for acne. This procedure was originally developed to treat facial scarring. Today these procedures are also used to reduce the appearance of facial lines and wrinkles, and to treat severe sun damage. Using a tool that looks like a dentist's drill, a dermatology surgeon will move the spinning wheel over the surface of the face. There are various sizes and grades of wheels that are used, depending on the objective of the surgery. Following dermabrasion, the skin will be red, swollen, and tender, and it typically takes seven to ten days for these side effects to subside. With microdermabrasion, crystals are used instead of the wheel. The tiny crystals sprayed on the skin remove surface layers, thereby correcting fine lines and superficial scars. Microdermabrasion is less invasive than dermabrasion, but multiple treatments may be necessary.

Laser resurfacing. Lasers emit high-intensity light to treat wrinkles and facial scars caused by acne, blemishes, and skin growths. The carbon dioxide from the lasers remove top layers of the skin with the goal of replacing old or damaged skin with new, evenly toned skin. This procedure is also called a *laser peel*. It can take one to four weeks to heal from laser surgery. Risks associated with laser resurfacing include burning, scarring, lightening (hypopigmentation) or darkening (hyperpigmentation) of the skin, and potential activation of infections such as the herpes virus (in the form of cold sores). A more gentle form of laser resurfacing is fraxel. Fraxel laser treatments have fewer side effects than other laser peels and only take a few days to heal.

Pulsed light. Light-emitting diode (LED), photomodulation, and intense pulsed light (IPL) use low-intensity pulsed light to promote circulation and healthy skin cell activity. The intensity is so low that heat is not emitted. It is typically used to reduce wrinkles, hyperpigmentation, redness, roughness, and pore size. Some research has shown that it can reverse signs of photoaging and may even be effective in some cases of early skin cancer. Pulsed light therapies can cause skin to turn pink and have the sensation of mild sunburn. In rare cases, bruising and hair loss may occur. You should avoid sun exposure for several days before and after the treatment. You can typically return to work immediately following pulsed light therapy.

Cosmetic surgery. Cosmetic surgery is an option for some individuals. Also known as plastic surgery, this category of treatment is extremely broad. Expensive surgical techniques can literally and completely change

---

DID YOU KNOW?

People who live to be one hundred are known as centenarians. It is estimated that there are more than seventy thousand people over the age of a hundred living in the United States, and centenarians are the fastest-growing age group. Compared to just twenty years ago, that's triple the number of one-hundred-plus-year-olds. According to Discover *magazine, "New data indicates that average human life expectancy is likely to reach 100 by the year 2060."*

the shape and look of your face. Be aware that these surgical procedures come with a myriad of risks and potential complications. Anti-aging plastic surgery focuses on the following areas:

- Collagen or fat injections to plump up creased, furrowed, or sunken facial skin and lips

- Eyelid surgery to lift drooping upper eyelids or remove excess fat, skin, and muscle under the eyes (often referred to as "bags")

- Facelift, which actually re-drapes the skin by removing the excess and tightens muscles to improve sagging skin on the face, jaw line, and neck

- Facial implants, which change the shape and balance of the face, typically focusing on the chin, cheekbones, and jaw line

- Forehead lift, which involves an incision (or more than one incision) just behind the hairline at the top of the head to remove excess tissue; this minimizes forehead creases and frown lines, drooping eyebrows, and hooding over the eyes

A wide array of side effects are associated with all plastic surgical procedures. One of the most common is scarring. According to plastic surgeon Simon Withey, MD, "Every day we will see people who have had problems from operations. In some cases you can do revisional surgery, but in some cases they are scarred for life." Dr. Withey described to BBC News several plastic surgery horror stories, including that of a woman who was supposed to have a simple eyelid surgery to tighten up the skin. "When I saw her she had a scar halfway up the lid and cheek," he told the BBC. "It was hideous."

Be sure to evaluate all the risks associated with the surgical procedure you are considering. Extra care and time should be taken before choosing plastic surgery as an option.

Fortunately, there are many things you can do without resorting to plastic surgery. Begin by looking at the topical products you are using and consider changing your present skin care routine. There are also specific yoga and Pilates moves that tone the facial and neck muscles, giving you a minilift. For more information on diet and exercise, see Chapter 9.

HEALTHY AGING INGREDIENTS

INGREDIENT	BENEFITS
Cloudberry seed oil	High in alpha linolenic acids, contains free vitamin E and its UV-protecting carotenoids and cell-membrane-strengthening phytosterols are found in abundance in the oil. Cloudberry seed oil offers a unique combination of energy and nutrition.
EGCG (green tea)	Exceptional antioxidant properties, which quench free radicals.
L-proline	An essential nutrient involved in the production of collagen; 21% of collagen is made up of L-proline.
L-sodium hyaluronate	The major constituent of collagen in the human body, this vegetarian source of hyaluronic acid is utilized by the skin to produce collagen; helps maintain the precious moisture balance in the skin.
Resveratrol (grapes)	Provides phenomenal antioxidant protection.
Thermous Thermophilus Ferment (aka Venuceane)	A powerful antioxidant. It protects against UV damage (lipoperoxidation, DNA and fibroblasts oxidation, skin enzyme inactivation).
Pisum Sativum (Pea) Extract (aka Proteasyl TP)	A peptide from Pisum sativum (Pea) protects and repairs epidermal proteins. Also protects against damage induced by proteases activated by environmental toxins (pollution, stress, UV, etc.).
L-ascorbic acid (10% concentration or higher)	Stimulates collagen production and fights free radicals.
Retinol	Retinol from carrots, cantaloupe, and sweet potatoes promotes cellular turnover and supports healing of the skin.
Acetyl Tetrapeptide-2 (Thymulen 4)	A peptide that induces an increase in keratins and keratohyalins in the stratum granulosum and boosts epidermis regeneration.
Palmitoyl tripeptide-3 (aka SYN-COLL)	A small peptide capable of stimulating collagen synthesis in human fibroblasts.
SYN-TACKS (Palmitoyl tripeptide diaminobutyloylhydroxythreonine, palmitoyl dipeptide diamino-hydroxybutyrate)	Increases formation of collagen and elastin and protects against moisture loss.

IT'S NEVER TOO LATE

The 76-plus million American baby boomers have made it quite clear—they are very interested in renewing their skin's youthful glow. They are "against" aging. But they also realize that certain aspects of aging are inevitable.

Reducing sun exposure and protecting the skin from the elements—especially damaging UV rays—is the first step on the path to younger-looking skin. Beyond that, to address aging skin, we must address the underlying causes while supporting and healing the entire infrastructure of the skin. This plan begins with effective, nontoxic, topical products that are incorporated into a consistent daily skin care routine. We can also use some medical treatments to get our skin on the right track.

One of the most important things to remember when it comes to healthy aging skin is that it's never too late! You can have healthier, younger-looking skin at any age—you just need to begin today.

Along the Journey

Aging in Arizona

Several years ago, I was doing a product demonstration at a major natural health store. Two sisters in their mid- to late forties approached me afterwards. As one of the women asked her question, I was looking at her skin—it's a habit I've picked up over the years. I answered her question and then I asked her, "Do you mind if I spray your face with this hydrating mist?"

"No, go ahead," she said. She waited a few seconds and said, "Oh, this is refreshing! Thank you." I could tell that her skin was severely dehydrated. She and her sister went shopping in the store and I continued to answer more questions from different customers.

About twenty minutes later, they returned, smiling. "Why did you spray me with that mist?" asked the one sister.

"I could tell that your skin was dehydrated and I knew that this mist would give you some relief."

"Well, it's amazing how much better my skin feels in such a short period of time. Tell me more about it!"

I began telling her about the dangers of dehydration and how spraying a mist that contains heavy water and fruit enzymes will help her sooth her dehydrated skin. I told her that it is especially important to use a mist in dry climates like Arizona or Colorado where I live. As I continued to talk about nourishing creams and other ways to help heal aging skin, a crowd gathered. I told them that quick fixes are not the answer and that we must look at the underlying causes of aging skin. Something as simple as remedying dehydration can make all the difference in the world. After I was done speaking, the woman gathered up several products, took one of my cards and went to the checkout line.

Two weeks later, I received a letter from her. She said she was shocked at how healthy and fresh her skin felt in just two weeks. She explained that people have even commented on her skin and asked what she was doing. She said that even her skeptical sister has been converted.

9

From the Inside Out

N̲ontoxic, effective skin care products are critical to achieving and maintaining healthy, vibrant skin. But while the skin may be a "surface" organ, which often responds to topical treatments, achieving and maintaining healthy skin requires us to consider the inside as well as the outside. It is irresponsible to simply promote products as skin-saving miracles and wrinkle cures without endorsing a healthy lifestyle that complements those products. If you want radiant, healthy-looking skin, you must address your skin care from the inside out. It's a package deal.

The skin is like a mirror for our internal organs and body systems, reflecting the status of our overall health. The opposite is also true: Our overall health can directly influence the health of our skin.

Extensive research has clearly demonstrated that a healthful diet, regular exercise, and other positive lifestyle factors can prevent a variety of diseases. What many people don't realize, however, is that the same principles will not only help fend off illness, they will also help you achieve the youthful skin you desire. Dealing with diet is a perfect place to start.

THE DIETARY CONNECTION

One of the most appropriate acronyms I have found is for the Standard American Diet (SAD). Yes, the standard diet for most Americans is very sad. According to an article by Mike Adams on Newstarget.com, Americans are getting nearly one-third of their calories from junk foods—soft drinks, sweets, desserts, alcoholic beverages, and salty snacks. "We are a nation of people who are simultaneously overfed and malnourished," reports Adams. "In other words, we're getting plenty of calories, but very little nutrition."

The typical North American diet is high in animal fats, low in fiber, high in processed foods, and low in plant-based foods. "The striking fact is that cultures that eat the reverse of the standard American diet—low fat, high in complex carbohydrates, plant-based, and high in fiber—have a lower incidence of cancer and coronary artery disease," explains William Sears, MD.

A study reported in the *New England Journal of Medicine* confirmed that

Top Ten Dietary Dos

Here's a list of foods that contain important, antioxidant-rich vitamins, minerals, flavonoids and other active compounds that can help enhance skin health. For younger, healthy-looking skin, add lots of these items to your daily diet:

1. Green Tea

2. Spinach and other leafy green vegetables

3. Colorful fruits, such as blueberries, grapes, and strawberries

4. Citrus fruits

5. Coldwater fish, such as salmon, halibut, and cod

6. Carrots, peppers, tomatoes, beets, and other colorful vegetables

7. Broccoli, cauliflower, and other cruciferous vegetables

8. Spices, especially turmeric, rosemary, and ginger

9. Pumpkin seeds, nuts, and whole grains

10. Garlic and onions

Top Ten Dietary and Lifestyle Don'ts

Here's a list of diet and lifestyle activities that should be avoided. Try to eliminate or reduce your practice or consumption of the following:

1. Smoking

2. Lack of exercise

3. Alcohol

4. Fried foods

5. Junk foods and "fast" foods

6. Stress

7. Lack of sleep

8. Foods with preservatives, additives, and artificial ingredients

9. Smoked and processed meats

10. Empty-calorie foods like candy, soft drinks, and chips

obesity, which is associated with the standard American diet, shortens our lives. According to the researchers, as you gain pounds, you will lose years.

In addition to length of life, we can easily link our diet to the development of certain illnesses, like heart disease, cancer, and diabetes. The same connection can be made with our skin. Our diet is not just linked to acne, as discussed in Chapter 6, it can influence every aspect of the health of our skin.

All cells of the human body—including our skin cells—need proper nourishment in order to thrive. As we learned in Chapter 1, skin cells are active. They are born, grow, and age, just as we do. The vitality of their short life span is determined not only by how we take care of them externally, but also by how we feed them internally. Because our skin is the largest organ of the body and skin cells are constantly being bombarded by external factors, we need to nourish them properly so they can withstand the test of time.

In addition to providing nourishment to skin cells, a healthy diet can also help reduce internal inflammation. Conversely, a poor diet can increase inflammation. Science has shown us that chronic internal and external inflammation can damage skin cells and cause us to age more rapidly. Typically, when we think of inflammation, we think of it from an external perspective, for example, in connection with an injury. However, there is also an internal process known as the *inflammatory response*. This is when the cells of our immune system respond to free radicals, which are dangerous molecules that damage cells. It is believed that free radical damage is a leading cause of accelerated aging and can contribute to many illnesses, including heart disease and cancer. Free radicals can also harm the skin.

A free radical is a molecule that has lost a piece of itself. It's like an airplane with only one wing. It spins out of control, looking for its missing wing trying to steal one from a healthy cell. A free radical tries to steal pieces from our healthy cells in an attempt to become whole again. In the process, it damages the cells it touches.

"Free radicals are in the air we breathe, the water we drink, and the foods we eat," according to the *Definitive Guide to Cancer*. "These reactive molecules can damage cells through oxidation, a destructive process similar to the way oxygen can cause rust, which can destroy a car."

Free radicals can also cause inflammation. Although free radicals are dangerous, they can be controlled by antioxidants in our food. The connection between diet and disease is clear: If our diet is poor, not only do we create more free radicals, but we also don't ingest enough antioxidants to eliminate those free radicals.

Over the past two and a half decades that I have been involved in the holistic industry, I have learned a wealth of information about the destructiveness of free radicals. Free radicals are involved in every aspect of aging, most visibly with the skin. This includes thinning of the skin, wrinkles, deep lines, sagging, hyperpigmentation, and loss of tone, texture, and vibrancy.

In addition to a poor diet, a variety of factors increase our exposure to free radicals, including smoking, stress, and pollution. Free radical damage is cumulative and can take years before we see its visible effects. The good news is that it's never too late to switch to a wrinkle-reducing, healthy diet.

The more antioxidants we absorb externally and internally, the better our chances of eradicating free radicals. In addition to the topical antioxidants discussed in previous chapters, foods also contain powerful antioxidants.

SKIN-FRIENDLY FOODS

There are foods that heal and foods that harm. The key is to choose the healing foods as much as possible. Special emphasis should be placed on fruits and vegetables.

When evaluating dietary choices, as explained in the previous section, it makes sense to choose foods that have antioxidant activity. Fortunately, many of those foods are easy to identify because they are colorful. Here is a general rule of thumb: If the foods on your dinner plate are void of color, you are not getting enough antioxidant nutrients. Be sure to add some color to your meals!

The vibrant colors of some foods come from a group of antioxidants known as flavonoids. The orange found in carrots and peppers, the red in tomatoes and ruby red trout, the green in spinach, the pink of the salmon, and the blue in blueberries are signaling that you have made the right choice. The more colorful your food, the better it is for you—and for your skin. Of course, the only exception to this rule is artificial colors, which are *not* good for you or your skin. I try to eat as many colorful fresh vegetables and fruits as I can, but if my life gets a bit hectic, I supplement my diet with a green superfood drink to get the antioxidant protection I need. The brands I prefer are Amazing Grass, Barleans, Garden of Life, or Udos.

We need to eat foods that are as close to their natural state as possible—just as nature intended. This will help ensure that the food contains the many vitamins, minerals, and other nutrients that our skin needs. Eat-

Four Key Dietary Supplements to Consider

Your dietary supplement plan should be individualized based on your diet and your health goals. I'm often asked to narrow the field and recommend just a few key dietary supplements. Here are four that I think are very important to most people and provide a solid foundation to build upon:

1. Multivitamin/mineral formula

2. Essential fatty acids (also referred to as fish oil supplements)

3. Probiotics (containing acidophilus and other beneficial bacteria)

4. An antioxidant formulation (should contain typical antioxidants, such as vitamins E and C, but also other antioxidants, such as resveratrol, green tea, and CoQ_{10})

In addition to these four key dietary supplements, there are also some dietary ingredients that are specifically beneficial to the skin. These include:

- Minerals, such as zinc and selenium

- Flavonoids from citrus and berries

- B vitamins, such as biotin, folic acid, and B_{12}

ing raw or lightly steamed vegetables is very important to get valuable nutrients like lycopene from tomatoes, lutein from carrots and peppers, and indole-3-carbinol from broccoli. Do not overcook vegetables because you will destroy the ingredients you need.

I recommend at least five servings of vegetables daily and at least two servings of fruit each day. This is not as difficult as it may sound when you consider that all of the items in the box on page 133 are considered to be one serving.

Incorporating colorful fruits and vegetables into your daily diet can be easier than you think. If you have a healthy salad that contains two cups of mixed leafy greens, half a cup of a variety of nonleafy vegetables (peppers,

---

Each of these represents one serving:

1 cup (240ml) raw leafy vegetables	$\frac{1}{2}$ cup (120ml) cut-up fruit
$\frac{1}{2}$ cup (120ml) raw nonleafy vegetables	1 cup (240ml) berries
$\frac{1}{2}$ cup (120ml) cooked vegetables	4 ounces (113g) 100% juice
$\frac{1}{2}$ cup (120ml) fresh vegetable juice	$\frac{1}{4}$ cup (60ml) dried fruit
1 medium fruit	

---

tomatoes, avocados, and broccoli are my favorite things to add to salads), some dried fruit, and some apple slices, you are nearly at the five-serving goal—and that's just one meal!

The next dietary component to focus on is fats. Believe it or not, there are actually "good" fats. These fats are called essential fatty acids (EFAs). Fats found in wild fish, nuts, seeds, and avocados are examples of good fats. Try substituting avocado for butter on toast—it's delicious! One of the reasons EFAs are considered good fats is that they actually help reduce internal inflammation. Omega-3 EFAs are especially beneficial and have been shown to prevent heart disease and cancer. Good dietary sources of omega-3s are flaxseeds, pumpkin seeds, sunflower seeds, walnuts, and green leafy vegetables. I eat lots of avocados for the healthy fat content.

Saturated fats and trans fats are the dangerous "bad" fats. Saturated fats are found in red meat, butter, cheese, whole milk, and cream. Saturated fat intake should be limited and, if you eat meat, you should always choose the leanest cut and only buy from organic and free-range companies that you can trust (for more information on vegetarian and vegan diets, visit www.farmsanctuary.com).

Trans fats are far more dangerous than any other type of fat because they have been shown to contribute to both heart disease and cancer. "These fats are so bad for the body that effective January 1, 2006, food manufacturers are required to list both saturated and trans fat amounts on the label," according to the *Definitive Guide to Cancer*. When consumers know the content of the type of fats they can choose from, they can more easily avoid foods that are high in trans fats. Some places in the United

States, such as New York City, have even banned trans fats from being used in restaurants. Avoid trans fats whenever possible.

Whole grains are also great for the skin because they help with digestion, detoxification, and elimination. Detoxification is our body's internal mechanism for getting rid of the toxins we are exposed to. The skin is the largest detoxifying organ in the body. Eating whole grains supports efficient detoxification and therefore, contributes to healthy skin.

Research from the University of Minnesota found in 2004 that the average American was eating less than one serving of whole grains daily. The USDA recommends at least three servings daily (see figure below). Good sources of whole grains include whole wheat bread, whole grain cereal, and whole grain pasta. One slice of whole wheat bread is considered a serving. So build a healthy sandwich that includes two slices of whole wheat bread and you are two-thirds of the way to your whole grain daily dietary goal.

The USDA Food Guide Pyramid

KEY: These symbols show fats, oils, and added sugars in foods

◯ Fats (Naturally occurring and added)
▽ Sugars (added)

Fats, Oils, & Sweets
Use sparingly

Milk, Yogurt, & Cheese Group
2–3 Servings

Meat, Poultry, Fish, Dry Beans, Eggs, & Nuts Group
2–3 Servings

Vegetable Group
3–5 Servings

Fruit Group
2–4 Servings

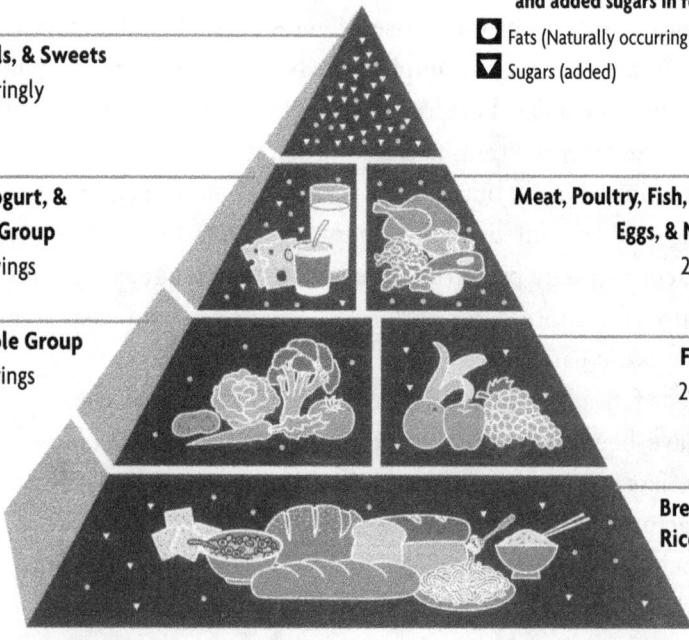

Bread, Cereal, Rice, & Pasta* Group
6–11 Servings

Sources: U.S. Department of Agriculture (www.mypyramid.gov) and U.S. Department of Health and Human Services
Whole grain products recommended.

As mentioned previously, I also endorse organic foods. I understand that organic foods may be a little more expensive and also hard to find in some communities; however, whenever you can, eat organic. As mentioned in the acne chapter, this is particularly important when it comes to dairy products. Also choose organic meat because it comes from animal sources that have not been given antibiotics or growth hormones. There are a variety of reasons why organic foods are a good choice. According to food scientist and writer Mary Mulry, PhD, many studies demonstrate that organic foods are higher in nutrients than conventionally grown foods and also contain far fewer toxins. Organic foods are produced without pesticides, synthetic fertilizers, supplemental hormones, antibiotics, genetic engineering, and they're not irradiated, meaning the soil they are grown in is not stripped of valuable nutrients.

"Organic standards in the United States are currently regulated by the U.S. Department of Agriculture," according to the *Definitive Guide to Cancer.* "These standards and the regulation of these standards continue to be hotly debated; however, we highly recommend choosing organic foods whenever possible."

In addition to eating organic, if you are taking dietary supplements, you are not alone. Harvard researcher David Eisenberg, MD, made headlines more than a decade ago when he released his findings that one-third of all Americans used alternative therapies. Most of those people were taking one or more dietary supplements. Follow-up studies by Dr. Eisenberg and other researchers have found that the percentage is even higher. Many Americans are using dietary supplements because they fear they are not getting enough nutrients through their diet—and they're right. Even for the most meticulous consumer, it is nearly impossible to get everything we need from food alone. Food processing, stress, the environment, and many other factors make dietary supplements a necessary part of our daily routine. Keep in mind, however, that dietary supplements should never take the place of healthy foods. As the name implies, these products are supplements to the diet. For a list of key supplements, see the inset on page 132.

Your diet can either help or harm your skin. By making smart dietary choices, you can dramatically increase your chances of having healthy, vibrant, younger-looking skin. When it comes to your skin, the most important lifestyle factor to focus on beyond diet is definitely consistent exercise.

GET PHYSICAL

That old Olivia Newton-John song "Let's Get Physical" should be our healthy skin mantra. There is clear scientific evidence that exercise is one of the most powerful, youth-promoting activities we can do.

However, for a long time, many of us thought that if we weren't wearing spandex and a matching sweatband we were not exercising. We now understand that movement—that is, physical activity—is medicine. It doesn't matter if you love to run, train with weights, bicycle, hike, ski, or just walk around the block. The key is to get moving.

"We all experience the gentle—and sometimes not so gentle—tug of aging," explains Susan Ryan, DO, a sports medicine specialist and emergency room physician at Rose Medical Center in Denver, Colorado. "Every physiologic system undergoes a gradual decline in its operational efficiencies. Although exercise does not prevent these changes in their entirety, it can certainly slow down the process."

I have always been aware of the direct benefit of exercising—maintaining a healthy weight. However, I have learned over the years that weight loss is just the tip of the exercise iceberg. When we are physically active, we experience a broad range of physiological benefits. Exercise can help:

- strengthen our immune system
- improve our mood and self-image
- increase energy levels
- improve circulation
- enhance detoxification
- reduce insomnia
- improve digestion

🦁 strengthen muscles and bone mass

🦁 balance hormones

Let's face it: There is no other medicine available that can do all that! Because exercise has such a positive influence on all of these key body systems, it's not surprising that it will also help our skin.

"In the long run, people who exercise have a better complexion overall," according to David Goldberg, MD, dermatologist and clinical professor of dermatology at Mt. Sinai Medical Center in New York City.

Two key ways that exercise directly and positively influences the health of our skin is through stress control and sweating. Regular exercise increases sweating, which helps unclog pores and reduces breakouts. According to David Berman, MD, former chief of dermatology at Santa Clara County Hospital in California, exercise helps control stress and by reducing stress we reduce hormone production. This is important because there is a direct link between hormone production and our skin, especially in the case of acne.

The connection between exercise and our skin goes even further. Exer-

DID YOU KNOW?

According to the National Institutes of Health, nearly two-thirds of the adult population is classified as obese, with a body mass index (BMI) greater than 30 (to calculate your BMI, refer to the chart on pages 138 and 139). Even worse, obesity among children is increasing at an alarming rate. The number of children aged six to eleven who were classified as overweight went from 6.5 percent in the late 1970s to nearly 19 percent in 2003–2004. For children aged twelve to nineteen, it shot up from 5 percent to more than 17 percent. Here's a great tip from author and naturopathic physician Dr. Lise Alschuler: "I tell my patients that they should be able to see the edges of their plate and stop eating when they are nearly full." Dr. Alschuler says that, in general, the size of our meal portions is too large. Bottom line: If you want super skin, don't "supersize" your meal!

cise keeps our skin looking youthful by enhancing collagen production. Remember, collagen is the connective tissue that keeps our skin looking plump and youthful. Collagen production diminishes as we age, making our skin dry and wrinkled. Exercise bathes the body in oxygen and also helps transport nutrients to skin cells. This is the perfect environment for healthy collagen production.

BODY MASS INDEX TABLE

	NORMAL						OVERWEIGHT					OBESE						
BMI:	19	20	21	22	23	24	25	26	27	28	29	30	31	32	33	34	35	36
HEIGHT	BODY WEIGHT (POUNDS)																	
58"	91	96	100	105	110	115	119	124	129	134	138	143	148	153	158	162	167	172
59"	94	99	104	109	114	119	124	128	133	138	143	148	153	158	163	168	173	178
60"	97	102	107	112	118	123	128	133	138	143	148	153	158	163	168	174	179	184
61"	100	106	111	116	122	127	132	137	143	148	153	158	164	169	174	180	185	190
62"	104	109	115	120	126	131	136	142	147	153	158	164	169	175	180	186	191	196
63"	107	113	118	124	130	135	141	146	152	158	163	169	175	180	186	191	197	203
64"	110	116	122	128	134	140	145	151	157	163	169	174	180	186	192	197	204	209
65"	114	120	126	132	138	144	150	156	162	168	174	180	186	192	198	204	210	216
66"	118	124	130	136	142	148	155	161	167	173	179	186	192	198	204	210	216	223
67"	121	127	134	140	146	153	159	166	172	178	185	191	198	204	211	217	223	230
68"	125	131	138	144	151	158	164	171	177	184	190	197	203	210	216	223	230	236
69"	128	135	142	149	155	162	169	176	182	189	196	203	209	216	223	230	236	243
70"	132	139	146	153	160	167	174	181	188	195	202	209	216	222	229	236	243	250
71"	136	143	150	157	165	172	179	186	193	200	208	215	222	229	236	243	250	257
72"	140	147	154	162	169	177	184	191	199	206	213	221	228	235	242	250	258	265
73"	144	151	159	166	174	182	189	197	204	212	219	227	235	242	250	257	265	272
74"	148	155	163	171	179	186	194	202	210	218	225	233	241	249	256	264	272	280
75"	152	160	168	176	184	192	200	208	216	224	232	240	248	256	264	272	279	287
76"	156	164	172	180	189	197	205	213	221	230	238	246	254	263	271	279	287	295

Adapted from *Clinical Guidelines on the Identification, Evaluation, and Treatment of Overweight and Obesity in Adults: The Evidence Report.*

Certain exercises can even help break up cellulite. "Stretching tones and conditions the muscles," says Vasanthi Bhat, founder of Vasantha Yoga Health and Fitness in Santa Clara, California. "Skin attached to those muscles becomes firm and beautiful." According to Bhat, practicing yoga every day is like getting a facelift. "Backward-bending poses, such as fish, camel, and cobra, have the power of a facelift, if done regularly, while forward-

BODY MASS INDEX TABLE																	
OBESE				EXTREME OBESITY													
BMI: 37	38	39	40	41	42	43	44	45	46	47	48	49	50	51	52	53	54
HEIGHT						BODY WEIGHT (POUNDS)											
58" 177	181	186	191	196	201	205	210	215	220	224	229	234	239	244	248	253	258
59" 183	188	193	198	203	208	212	217	222	227	232	237	242	247	252	257	262	267
60" 189	194	199	204	209	215	220	225	230	235	240	245	250	255	261	266	271	276
61" 195	201	206	211	217	222	227	232	238	243	248	254	259	264	269	275	280	285
62" 202	207	213	218	224	229	235	240	246	251	256	262	267	273	278	284	289	295
63" 208	214	220	225	231	237	242	248	254	259	265	270	278	282	287	293	299	304
64" 215	221	227	232	238	244	250	256	262	267	273	279	285	291	296	302	308	314
65" 222	228	234	240	246	252	258	264	270	276	282	288	294	300	306	312	318	324
66" 229	235	241	247	253	260	266	272	278	284	291	297	303	309	315	322	328	334
67" 236	242	249	255	261	268	274	280	287	293	299	306	312	319	325	331	338	344
68" 243	249	256	262	269	276	282	289	295	302	308	315	322	328	335	341	348	354
69" 250	257	263	270	277	284	291	297	304	311	318	324	331	338	345	351	358	365
70" 257	264	271	278	285	292	299	306	313	320	327	334	341	348	355	362	369	376
71" 265	272	279	286	293	301	308	315	322	329	338	343	351	358	365	372	379	386
72" 272	279	287	294	302	309	316	324	331	338	346	353	361	368	375	383	390	397
73" 280	288	295	302	310	318	325	333	340	348	355	363	371	378	386	393	401	408
74" 287	295	303	311	319	326	334	342	350	358	365	373	381	389	396	404	412	420
75" 295	303	311	319	327	335	343	351	359	367	375	383	391	399	407	415	423	431
76" 304	312	320	328	336	344	353	361	369	377	385	394	402	410	418	426	435	443

bending poses, such as child pose, bowing pose, and modified headstand, bring a rich blood supply to facial skin."

Other experts agree that exercise does not just loosen tight muscles, it also releases tension in the muscles—including the muscles of the face—creating toned skin. According to Dr. Goldberg, "Eventually, crow's feet and anger expression lines are going to soften up. Certainly you will prevent new ones from forming. So in this respect, regular exercise can help you look younger longer."

Have you ever noticed that people who exercise consistently have a healthier glow to their skin? That's because of improved circulation and detoxification. Ashen or gray skin can become pink and rosy with consistent exercise. Exercise enhances circulation by delivering valuable blood and oxygen to the skin cells while it simultaneously helps remove internal and external toxins we have been exposed to.

It's clear that exercise will help enhance the health of your skin and keep you looking and feeling younger. Here are some general exercise tips:

🐾 **Stay hydrated.** Drink plenty of water before, during, and after physical activity, especially if you are exercising in hot weather.

🐾 **Don't rush it.** If you haven't been active in a while, start gradually and increase the time and intensity as you can. You may need to see your doctor before embarking on a new exercise program. If you haven't exercised before, you may want to start out with twenty to thirty minutes of walking five days a week.

🐾 **Step it up.** After your initial workout becomes easier, increase the intensity, duration, or frequency. Forty-five minutes or more of moderate to vigorous activity five days a week is an excellent goal.

🐾 **Vary your routine.** To stay interested in exercise, don't be afraid to mix it up with a few activities that you really enjoy. A varied exercise routine is easier to stick with over the long term.

🐾 **Make it a way of life.** Make a commitment to adding exercise to your regular routine. Being physically active should be a way of life.

Exercise is also a great way to reduce stress, which will also benefit the skin. When I get a bit overwhelmed or I am feeling stressed, I take a short walk. Even just a ten- minute walk can make a world of difference. Remember to always cleanse your face following intense exercise. This will remove sweat, dead cells, and other debris that surfaced during your workout.

THE MIND MATTERS

Not that long ago, scientists believed there was no direct connection between mind and body, that the two were not only separate entities but also independent of each other. Today, we recognize that just the opposite is true: Mind, body, and spirit are intimately connected and irrefutably dependent on one another.

Mind-body-spirit medicine (also known as holistic, integrative, or complementary medicine) has garnered tremendous news coverage in recent years and has been embraced by a majority of the population. While this entire realm is fascinating to me, I have lumped the mind-body-spirit issues that are most significant into three categories:

1. Stress reduction

2. Love, support, and spirituality

3. The power of positive thinking

Chronic stress that becomes unmanageable has clearly been linked to serious illnesses, such as cancer and heart disease. In addition to accelerating the overall aging process, chronic stress can also damage the skin. The most visible signs of this are worry lines and wrinkles.

Stress is part of our daily lives, and not all stress is bad. Stress helps us meet our deadlines, finish the race, or run from a mugger. This is known as the fight-or-flight response that is hardwired into each one of us. But when the stress is incessant and our bodies begin to physically change based on our daily exposure to stress, we have a problem. We are no longer running from a mugger, we are just getting through the day. Our internal environment is wound tight, just like the frowns on our faces.

There are a variety of relaxation techniques that can help us alleviate our stress and loosen those frown lines. Meditation, breathing exercises, yoga, massage, and other activities are designed to help us deal with stress. But we can also alleviate stress by reading, walking in the park, or listening to music. The key is to create an individualized stress reduction program that works for you. Tackle your stress head on. If you try to ignore your stress, you will see the damage it can cause gazing back at you in the mirror.

I am very fortunate to have the love and support of family and friends. My husband and daughter are gifts in my life that help me experience joy and happiness every day. My two sisters are also very special to me. They support and nurture me during challenging times and share in my happiness as well. The love I receive from my family—and the love I return to them—actually enhances my health.

"Numerous studies have linked healthy companionship, support groups, and fulfilling relationships to overall well-being, survival, and quality of life," according to Lise Alschuler, ND, coauthor of the *Definitive Guide to Cancer*. "Our relationships and how we connect with others can provide a rich dimension to our lives and to our healing process."

Spirituality and connecting with a higher power or something beyond ourselves is also an important component in the mind-body connection. Spirituality transcends religious denominations, although it certainly can entail religious practices, such as prayer. The way I connect to my spiritual being is by giving back to society through my volunteer work and my contributions to my community. To me, spirituality can be reflected in our willingness to give. It's not important how you define spirituality, but it is important how you connect with your spiritual being. To enhance the mind-body connection, be sure to focus on the spiritual aspect as well.

I have been told that I am a very positive person. I have studied the power of positive thinking for decades and incorporated some of its concepts into both my personal and professional lives. By focusing on emotions, such as joy and happiness, as well as vibrant health, success, and peace, we can be receptive to actually receiving the positive feelings we cultivate. I'm not advocating the creation of a false sense of exuberance no matter what the circumstance. It's important to be authentic in expressing how we feel.

"Sadness can bring you down into the depths of your own inner ocean, where treasures often lie," eloquently explains Dr. Alschuler. "You need to occasionally dive down there to gather those riches. The key is to come back up before you run out of air and then to use what you have found to enrich your life experience at the surface."

Just as your exterior is a reflection of your physical inner health, it also reflects the connection you are making between mind, body, and spirit. Making that connection will help you not only achieve vibrant, youthful skin, but also experience the joy and happiness that can come with a truly integrative health program.

IT'S A WRAP—YOUR WRAP!

We are what we eat, think, and feel. How we balance work, stress, relationships, and fun contributes to our overall health and the health of our skin. Making conscious decisions every day will lead to a more fulfilled life. But remember, nobody's perfect. If you get off track, don't be too hard on yourself. After all, we're only human.

Throughout this book, I have spelled out practical things that can help you have the skin you desire. Hopefully, you have learned that you have the power to take control of your skin and your overall health in the process. For some, it will not be an easy journey, but your persistence and dedication will pay off.

Don't be intimidated by the demands of your skin. I am a firm believer in the 80/20 rule. Very few of us can live completely healthy lives 100 percent of the time. Instead of berating myself when I falter, I remind myself that I make healthy choices 80 percent of the time and allow myself to indulge 20 percent. The healthy choices become second nature as we make them more a part of our daily routines. When we look in the mirror, our skin tells us if we are on the right track.

If you have wonderful skin, you can maintain its vibrancy for years to come with a comprehensive, individualized approach. You can use that same plan to transform your skin and achieve the youthful radiance you are looking for. Skin care requires a thorough health-promoting program, featuring a healthful diet, lots of physical activity, and a positive mind-body approach to life. Beyond the basics, healthy skin for a lifetime will only come from using nontoxic, yet effective skin care products. It's not only the right decision for your skin, it's the right thing to do for our environment.

Setting a higher standard in skin care begins with consumer choice. We must expose the dark side of the skin care industry so we can make informed, conscious choices about the products we apply to our skin. The power of our pocketbooks will dictate the change that is necessary in an industry that has been irresponsible for decades.

Selected References

CHAPTER 1

Alschuler Lise, & Karolyn A. Gazella. *Definitive Guide to Cancer: An Integrative Approach to Prevention, Treatment, and Healing.* Berkeley, Calif.: Celestial Arts, 2007.

Gambino, Henry J. *Modern Esthetics: A Scientific Source for Estheticians.* Albany, N.Y.: Melady, 1992.

Murray, Michael T. *Encyclopedia of Nutritional Supplements.* New York: Prima Publishing, 1996.

Niederdeppe J., & A. G. Levy. "Fatalistic Beliefs about Cancer and Three Prevention Behaviors." *Cancer Epidemiology Biomarkers Prevention* 16, no. 5 (May 2007): 998–1003.

Pierce, J. P., et al. "Greater Survival after Breast Cancer in Physically Active Woman with High Vegetable-Fruit Intake Regardless of Obesity." *Journal of Clinical Oncology* 25, no 17 (June 2007): 2345–2351.

Schwarz, T. "Skin Immunity." *British Journal of Dermatology* 149, no. s66 (November 2003): 2–4.

Website

U.S. National Institutes of Health: http://ods.od.nih.gov/factsheets/vitamind.asp

CHAPTER 2

Bergfeld, W. F., D. V. Belsito, J. G. Marks, & F. A. Andersen. "Safety Ingredients Used in Cosmetics." *Journal of the American Academy of Dermatology* 52, no. 1 (January 2005): 125–132.

Byford, J. R., et al. "Oestrogenic Activity of Parabens in mcf7 Human Breast Cancer Cells." *Journal of Steroid Biochemistry and Molecular Biology* 80, no. 1 (January 2002): 49–60.

EPA Executive Summary: The National Biennial RCRA Hazardous Waste Report (Based on 1995 Data), August 1997, published by the Environmental Protection Agency, Washington, D.C.

Erickson, Kim. *Drop-Dead Gorgeous: Protecting Yourself from the Hidden Dangers of Cosmetics.* New York: Contemporary Books, 2002.

Faroon, O., D. Jones, & C. de Rosa. "Effects of Polychlorinated Biphenyls on the Nervous System." *Toxicology and Industrial Health* 16, no. 7–8 (September 2001): 305–333.

Fred Hutchinson Cancer Research Center Newsletter. "Cook Study Suggests Link Between Ovarian Cancer, Genital Powders, Sprays." Seattle, April 3, 1997.

Gaynor, Mitchell. *Nurture Nature Nurture Health: Your Health and the Environment.* New York: Nurture Nature Press, 2005.

Guenther, K., V. Heinke, B. Thiele, E. Kleist, H. Prast, & T. Raecker. "Endocrine Disrupting Nonylphenols Are Ubiquitous in Food." *Environmental Science and Technology* 36 (2002): 1676–1680.

Kiely, T., D. Donaldson, & A. Grube. "Pesticides Industry Sales and Usage: 2000 and 2001 Market Estimates." U.S. Environmental Protection Agency, Washington, D.C., May 2004.

Lee, D. H., D. R. Jacobs, & M. Porta. "Association of Serum Concentrations of Persistent Organic Pollutants with the Prevalence of Learning Disability and Attention Deficit Disorder." *Journal of Epidemiology and Community Health* 61, no. 7 (2007): 591–596.

Lee, D. H., M. Steffes M, & D. R. Jacobs. "Positive Association of Serum Concentrations of Polychlorinated Biphenyls or Organochlorine Pesticides with Self-Reported Arthritis, Especially Rheumatoid Type, in Women." *Environmental Health Perspectives* 115, no. 6 (2007): 883–888.

Lee, D. H., et al. "Association between Serum Concentrations of Persistent Organic Pollutants and Insulin Resistance among Nondiabetic Adults: Results from the National Health and Nutrition Examination Survey 1999–2002." *Diabetes Care* 30, no. 3 (2007): 622–628.

National Toxicology Program. "NTP Toxicology and Carcinogenesis Studies of Chloroprene (CAS No. 126-99-8) in F344/N Rats and B6C3F1 Mice (Inhalation Studies)." National Toxicology Program Technical Report Series 467 (September 1998): 1–379.

Okubo. T., Y. Yokoyama, K. Kano, & I. Kano. "ER-Dependent Estrogenic Activity of Parabens Assessed by Proliferation of Human Breast Cancer MCF-7Cells and Expression of ER Alpha and PR." *Food and Chemical Toxicology* 39, no. 12 (December 2001): 1225–1232.

Pederson, K., et al. "The Preservatives Ethyl-, Propyl-, and Butylparaben Are Oestrognic in an In Vivo Fish Assay." *Pharmacological Toxicology* 86, no. 3 (2000): 110–113.

Roach, John. "Synthetic Fragrances Harmful to Marine Life, Study Says." *National Geographic News* (July 11, 2005).

Routledge, E. J., et al. "Some Alkyl Hydroxy Benzoate Preservatives (Parabens) Are Estrogenic." *Toxicology and Applied Pharmacology* 153, no. 1 (November 1998): 12–19.

Scanlan, R. A. "Nitrosamines and Cancer." The Linus Pauling Institute, 2000, Corvalis, Ore.

United Nations Environmental Programme (UNEP). "Chemicals, Inventory of Information Sources on Chemicals: Persistent Organic Pollutants." November 1999.

Websites

Food and Drug Administration: www.cfsan.fda.gov/~lrd/dioxinqa.html#g2

United Nations Environmental Programme: www.chem.unep.ch/pops/

www.cosmeticsdatabase.com/ingredient.php?ingred06=701828&refurl=/
company.php?comp_id=383&&nothanks=1

Environmental Working Group: www.ewg.org/reports/bodyburden/es.php/

Environmental Protection Agency (EPA): www.epa.gov/opfead1/international/
pops.htm • www.epa.gov/pcb/pubs/effects.html

Canadian Environmental Health Association: www.lesstoxicguide.ca/
index.asp?fetch=usage

Organic Consumers Association: www.organicconsumers.org/bodycare/ocalist090604.cfm

Cancer Prevention Coalition: www.preventcancer.com/consumers/cosmetics/talc.htm

CHAPTER 3

Gaynor, Mitchell. *Nurture Nature Nurture Health: Your Health and the Environment.* New York: Nurture Nature Press, 2005.

Gazella, Karolyn A. "Horse As Teacher." *Elephant* (Winter 2006/2007): 34–35.

Goldberg, A. M. "Animals and Alternatives: Societal Expectations and Scientific Need." *Alternatives to Laboratory Animals* 32, no. 6 (December 2004): 545–551.

James, Kat. *The Truth About Beauty: Transforming Your Looks and Your Life from the Inside Out.* Hillsboro, Ore.: Beyond Words Publishing, 2003.

"New! Misleading Product Claims." *Cosmetics & Toiletries* (May 30, 2006).

Rusche, B. "The 3Rs and Animal Welfare—Conflict or the Way Forward?" *Altex* 20, Supplement 1 (2003): 63–76.

Winter, R. *A Consumer's Dictionary of Cosmetic Ingredients.* New York: Three Rivers Press, 1999.

Yussefi, M., H. Willer, and B. Geier. "Organic Agriculture Worldwide: Still on the Rise in 2004." *Ecology and Farming* (January–April 2004): 12–14.

Websites

All for Animals: www.allforanimals.com/alternatives1.htm

British Broadcasting Company: www.bbc.co.uk/print/science/hottopics/animalexperiments/print.shtml

People for the Ethical Treatment of Animals (PETA): http://caringconsumer.com

Center for Food Safety & Applied Nutrition, U.S. Food and Drug Administration: www.cfsan.fda.gov/

Environmental Working Group: www.ewg.org/reports/skindeep2/findings

Humane Society of the United States: www.hsus.org/animals_in_research/animal_testing/

Medicine Horse: www.medicinehorse.org

Organic Trade Association: www.ota.com/definition/nosb.html • www.ota.com/definition/quickoverview.html

U.S. National Library of Medicine: www.ncbi.nlm.nih.gov/sites/ entrez?db=PubMed

U.S. National Institutes of Health (NIH): http://toxtown.nlm.nih.gov/ index_content.html

CHAPTER 4

Choi, C. M., & D. S. Berson. "Cosmeceuticals." *Seminars in Cutaneous Medicine and Surgery* 25, no. 3 (September 2006): 163–168.

Cosmeceuticals: Active Skin Treatment. Carol Stream, Ill.: Allured Publishing Corporation, 2002.

Currin, Morag. Personal correspondence, August 2007. See www.touchforcancer online.com.

Fitzpatrick, R. E., & E. F. Rostan. "Double-Blind, Half-Face Study Comparing Topical Vitamin C and Vehicle for Rejuvenation of Photodamage." *Dermatologic Surgery* 28, no. 3 (March 2002): 231–236.

Fraser, Jessica. "The Top Five Foods for Healthy Skin." NewsTarget.com, accessed September 13, 2006.

Harish, D., D. Kaushik, M. Gupta, V. Kumar, & V. Lather. "Cosmeceuticals: An Emerging Concept." *Indian Journal of Pharmacology* 37, no. 3 (July 2005): 155–159.

Jackson, E. M. "Assessing the Bioactivity of Cosmetic Products and Ingredients." *Skin Pharmacology and Applied Skin Physiology* 12, no. 3(May–June 1999): 125–131.

Kligman, A. M. "A Dermatologist Looks to the Future: Promises and Problems." *Dermatologic Clinics* 18, no. 4 (October 2000): 699–709.

Kuttalingam Gopalasubramaniam, S. Personal correspondence, August 2007.

Pilla, Louis. "Cosmetic vs Medical Dermatology: A Widening Gap?" *Skin & Aging* 11, no. 6 (June 2003): 32–37.

Traikovich, S. S. "Use of Topical Ascorbic Acid and its Effects on Photodamaged Skin Topography." *Archives of Otolaryngology—Head & Neck Surgery* 125, no. 10 (October 1999): 1091–1098.

CHAPTER 5

Baumann, Leslie. *The Skin Solution*. New York: Bantam Books, 2007.

Bevins, C. L., & F. T. Liu. "Rosacea: Skin Innate Immunity Gone Awry?" *Nature Medicine* 13 (2007): 904–906.

Currin, Morag. Personal interview, August 2007. See www.touchforcancer online.com.

Gambino, Henry J. *Modern Esthetics: A Scientific Source for Estheticians*. Albany, N.Y.: Milady, 1992.

Mature Market Institute of Met Life. "Demographic Profile: American Baby Boomers." Based on 2007 projections.

Wesley, N. O., & H. I. Maibach. "Racial (Ethnic) Differences in Skin Properties: The Objective Data." *American Journal of Clinical Dermatology* 4, no. 12 (2003): 843–860.

Websites

Website of Paula Begoun: www.cosmeticscop.com/learn/pf.asp?ID=40

Holistic Health Information: www.1stholistic.com/Beauty/skin/ skin_sensitive.htm

National Rosacea Society: www.rosacea.org

CHAPTER 6

Adebamowo, C. A., et al. "Milk Consumption and Acne in Adolescent Girls." *Dermatology Online Journal* 12, no. 4 (May 2006).

———. "High School Dietary Dairy Intake and Teenage Acne." *Journal of the American Academy of Dermatology* 52, no. 2 (February 2005): 207–214.

Farrar, M. D., & E. Ingham. "Acne: Inflammation." *Clinical Dermatology* 22, no. 5 (September–October 2004): 380–384.

Harper, J. C., & D. M. Thiboutot. "Pathogenesis of Acne: Recent Research Advances." *Advances in Dermatology* 19 (2003): 1–10.

Katzman, M., & A. C. Logan. "Acne Vulgaris: Nutritional Factors May Be Influencing Psychological Sequelae." *Medical Hypotheses* (April 2007): 1080–1084.

Leyden, J. J., et al. "Topical Retinoids in Inflammatory Acne: A Retrospective,

Investigator-Blinded, Vehicle-Controlled, Photographic Assessment." *Clinical Therapeutics* 27, no. 2 (February 2005): 216–224.

Lloyd, J. R. "The Use of Microdermabrasion for Acne: A Pilot Study." *Dermatology Surgery* 27, no. 4 (April 2001): 329–331.

Micol, V., et al. "Effects of Totarol, a Diterpenoid Antibacterial Agent, on Phospholipids Model Membranes." *Biochim Biophys Acta* 1511, no. 2 (April 2001): 281–290.

Murray, Michael T. *Natural Alternative to Over-the-Counter and Prescription Drugs.* New York: William Morrow & Company, 1994.

Thiboutot, D. "New Treatments and Therapeutic Strategies for Acne." *Archives of Family Medicine* 9, no. 2 (February 2000): 179–187.

Zaenglein, A. L., & D. M. Thiboutot. "Expert Committee Recommendations for Acne Management." *Pediatrics* 118, no. 3 (September 2006): 1188–1199.

Websites

Acne Resouce Center Online: www.acne-resource.org/understanding-acne/acne-statistics.html

Mayo Clinic: www.mayoclinic.com/health/antibiotics/FL00075

American Society of Plastic Surgeons: www.plasticsurgery.org/patients_consumers/procedures/Microdermabrasion.cfm

Website of Ray Sahleian, M.D.: www.raysahleian.com/acne.html

American Academy of Dermatology: www.skincarephysicians.com/acnenet/treatment.html

Mende Biotech Ltd.: www.totarol.com

CHAPTER 7

Alschuler, Lise, & Karolyn A. Gazella. *Definitive Guide to Cancer: An Integrative Approach to Prevention, Treatment, and Healing.* Berkeley, Calif.: Celestial Arts, 2007.

Barrow, Mary Mills, & John Barrows. *Sun Protection for Life.* Oakland, Calif.: New Harbinger Publications Inc., 2005.

Dal, H., et al. "Does Relative Melanoma Distribution of Body Size 1960–2004 Reflect Changes in Intermittent Exposure and Intentional Tanning in the

Swedish Population?" *European Journal of Dermatology* 17, no. 5 (August 2, 2007): 428–434. Print publication #17673388.

Wright, T. I., J. M. Spencer, & F. P. Flowers. "Chemoprevention of Non-melanoma Skin Cancer." *Journal of the American Academy of Dermatology* 54, no. 6 (2006): 933–46.

Websites

Environmental Protection Agency: www.epa.gov/sunwise/uvradiation.html

High Altitude Observatory at the University Corporation for Atmospheric Research: www.hao.ucar.edu/Public/education/basic.html

Sun Precautions, Inc.: www.sunprecautions.com/

CHAPTER 8

Alaluf, S., U. Heinrich, W. Stahl, H. Tronnier, & S. Wiseman S. "Dietary Carotenoids Contribute to Normal Human Skin Color and UV Photosensitivity." *Journal of Nutrition* 132, no. 3 (March 2002): 399–403.

Chertow, D. S., et al. "Botulism in 4 Adults Following Cosmetic Injections with an Unlicensed, Highly Concentrated Botulinum Preparation." *Journal of the American Medical Association* 296, no. 20 (November 22, 2006): 2476–2479.

Day, Doris J. *Forget the Facelift: Turn Back the Clock With a Revolutionary Program for Ageless Skin.* New York: Penguin Group, 2006.

Egawa, M., M. Oguri, T Kuwahara, & M. Takahashi. "Effect of Exposure of Human Skin to a Dry Environment." *Skin Research and Technology* 8, no. 4 (November 2002): 212–218.

Elliott, Jane. "Do Not Rush into Cosmetic Surgery." BBC News, October 29, 2004.

Holck, D. E., & J. D. Ng. "Facial Skin Rejuvenation." *Current Opinion in Ophthalmology* 14, no. 5 (October 2003): 246–252.

Leung, A. K., K. Keyhani, & M. Ashenhurst. "Retinal Tear and Raised Intraocular Pressure Following Unintentional Intraocular Botulium Toxin Type A Injection." *Canadian Journal of Ophthalmology* 42, no. 5 (October 2007): 746–747.

Purba, M. B., et al. "Skin Wrinkling: Can Food Make a Difference?" *Journal of the American College of Nutrition* 20, no. 1 (February 2001): 71–80.

Singer, Natasha. "Wrinkle Rivals Go to War." *New York Times* (Nov. 9, 2006).

Spencer, J. M. "Microdermabrasion." *American Journal of Clinical Dermatology* 6, no. 2 (2005): 89–92.

Weiss, R. A., et al. "Clinical Experience with Light-Emitting Diode (LED) Photomodulation." *Dermatologic Surgery* 31(9 Pt 2) (Sept 2005): 1199–1205.

Wright, Karen. "Staying Alive." *Discover* (November 6, 2003).

Websites

U.S. Centers for Disease Control (CDC): www.cdc.gov/ncidod/dbmd/ diseaseinfo/botulism_g.htm

New Zealand Dermatological Society: http://dermnetnz.org/site-age-specific/ wrinkles.html

Reliant Technologies: www.fraxel.com/

Humane Society of the United States: www.hsus.org/animals_in_research/ animals_in_research_news/hsus_files_complaint_against_fda.html

Mayo Clinic: www.mayoclinic.com/print/wrinkles/DS00890

National Institute of Aging, National Institutes of Health: www.nia.nih.gov/ NewsAndEvents/PressReleases/PR19990616NewCensus.htm

American Society of Plastic Surgeons: www.plasticsurgery.org/patients_ consumers/procedures/CosmeticPlasticSurgery.cfm

Science Daily: www.sciencedaily.com/releases/2007/02/070205232040.htm

CHAPTER 9

Alschuler Lise, and Karolyn A. Gazella. *Definitive Guide to Cancer: An Integrative Approach to Prevention, Treatment, and Healing.* Berkeley, Calif.: Celestial Arts, 2007.

Mulry, Mary, & Lara Evans Bracciante. "Why Organics? Understanding the Implications of Food Choices." *Health Reports* (March 29, 2005).

Murray, Michael T. *Natural Alternatives to Over-the-Counter and Prescription Drugs,*. New York: William Morrow & Company, 1994.

Murray, Michael T., Joseph Pizzorno, and Lara Pizzorno. *The Encyclopedia of Healing Foods.* New York: Atria Books, 2005.

Olashansky, S. J., et al. "A Potential Decline in Life Expectancy in the United

States in the 21st Century." *New England Journal of Medicine* 352, no. 11 (March 2005): 1138–1145.

Ryan, Susan. Personal interview, September 10, 2007.

Thompson, H. J., et al. "Effect of Increased Vegetable and Fruit Consumption on Markers of Oxidative Cellular Damage." *Carcinogenesis* 20, no. 12 (1999): 2261–2266.

Tindle, H. A., et al. "Trends in Use of Complementary and Alternative Medicine by U.S. Adults: 1997–2002." *Alternative Therapies in Health and Medicine* 11, no. 1 (2005): 42–49.

Websites

Website of Jim Sears, M.D.: www.askdrsears.com

U.S. Centers for Disease Control:
www.cdc.gov/nccdphp/dnpa/obesity/index.htm

News Target: www.newstarget.com/001109.html

Weight-Control Information Network, National Institutes of Health:
http://win.niddk.nih.gov/statistics/index.htm

USA Today: www.usatoday.com/news/health/2006-12-04-trans-fat-ban_x.htm

WebMD: www.webmd.com/skin-beauty/guide/exercise-your-body-your-skin

APPENDIX A

Skin Care Terms

acne vulgaris: medical term for acne, which is characterized by one or more blackheads, whiteheads, papules, or pustules

alpha hydroxy acid (AHA): fruit acid that helps slough off dead skin cells and encourages skin cell regeneration

basal layer: bottom layer of the epidermis, where new cells are continually produced

blackhead: noninflammatory acne lesions filled with excess oil and dead skin cells; also known as comedones

carcinoma: malignant cancerous tumor

bioactive ingredients: substances that cause physical changes and appearance

collagen: protein in skin tissue that contributes to the skin's elasticity

dermatitis: inflammation of the upper layers of the skin that can cause itching, blisters, and swelling

dermatology: the medical study of the skin and diseases that affect the skin

dermis: thick layer of the skin that contains blood, lymph vessels, sweat glands and nerve endings beneath the epidermis, the outermost layer of the skin

eczema: a skin disorder that involves inflammation of the upper layers of the skin; characterized by redness, swelling, itching, and dryness

elastin: a protein in connective tissue that is elastic

emollient: cream or lotion to help make the skin softer and smoother

epidermis: outermost layer of the skin; made up of five layers

exfoliant: product used to remove dead skin cells from the skin's surface

follicle: tiny shaft in the skin where hair grows and oil is secreted from the sebaceous glands

humectant: product that enhances moisture retention in the skin

hydration: bringing more water into skin tissues

hyperpigmentation: skin color that is darker than normal; caused by a number of factors, including, inflammation, sun damage, and acne

hyperthermia (also referred to as *heat stroke*): a heat-related illness typically caused by excess heat exposure

hypothermia (also referred to as *frostbite*): when body temperature drops below that which is required to function

melanin: dark brown or black skin pigment, naturally present in varying degrees

melanocytes: cells, located in the bottom layer of the skin's epidermis, which produce melanin, or skin pigment

melasma: patches of tan or dark facial discoloration, typically affecting women who are pregnant, taking oral contraceptives, or undergoing hormone replacement therapy; probably due to hormonal shifts that are affected by sun exposure

papule: inflammatory acne that looks like a small, red, raised bump on the skin

propionium bacteria (*P bacteria*): the bacteria that causes acne

psoriasis: a disease that affects skin and joints; commonly characterized by red, scaly patches and areas of inflammation that have a silvery-white appearance, due to excessive skin cell production

pustule: inflammatory acne that looks like a whitehead, due to pus formation in the top layer of the skin

rosacea: red, acnelike appearance on the face

sebaceous glands: glands located in the skin that produce sebum, an oily substance; these glands are attached to hair follicles and primarily located on the face, neck, back, and chest

sebum: an oily substance produced by the sebaceous glands in the skin

stratum basale: the deepest layer of the epidermis

stratum corneum: the outermost layer of the epidermis; made up mostly of dead skin cells

stratum granulosum: the layer of the epidermis that lies between the stratum spinosum and the stratum licidum

stratum licidum: the thin, clear layer of dead skin cells in the epidermis

stratum spinosum: the layer of epidermis that lies beneath the stratum granulosum

sun protection factor (SPF): a numerical system used to determine the effectiveness of sun-blocking products; the higher the number, the greater the protection from harmful ultraviolet rays from the sun

ultraviolet rays: radiation from the sun, which makes exposed skin become darker

viscosity: the liquidity and thickness of a solution

whitehead: a noninflammatory acne lesion where oil and dead skin cells block the opening of the hair follicle, also known as a closed comedone

APPENDIX B

Nourishing Ingredients

AC-Dermapeptide MicroC (saccharomyces/capsicum annum fruit ferment filtrate peptide): promotes collagen synthesis and circulation, and has anti-irritant properties; derived from red pepper or Capsicum annum

AC-Dermapeptide revitalizing (oriza sativa [rice] peptide): promotes cellular proliferation and regeneration, and has moisture-retention properties; derived from rice proteins

aesculus hippocastanum seed extract (horse chestnut) (HCE): exerts several beneficial effects on the circulatory system: tones the veins and helps reduce fluid accumulation in the tissues; also helps protect blood vessels from damaging free radicals and promotes circulation; promotes toning and acts as an astringent; reduces the permeability of capillaries and helps fragile and broken ones naturally

allantoin: See *symphytum officinale*

aloe vera barbadensis (aloe vera): a hydrating, softening, healing emollient with antimicrobial and anti-inflammatory properties

alpha hydroxy acids (AHAs): a family of naturally occurring acids with the ability to loosen binders holding dead skin cells together, thereby accelerating exfoliation of the stratum corneum

ananas comosus fruit extract (pineapple): contains bromelain, a keratin- (protein-) digesting enzyme

antarcticine: See *pseudoalteromas ferment extract*

antarctic seaweed: See *macrocystis pyrifera extract*

anthocyanins: powerful antioxidants from pigments found in berries

aminoguanidine: inhibits cross-linking of collagen (that is, it keeps the skin soft and pliable); from turnip juice, mushrooms, corn germ, and rice hulls

Applephenon™: See *pyrus malus fruit extract (apple)*

arnica montana (also known as leopard's bane, wolf's bane, mountain tobacco, and mountain arnica): reduces puffiness and swelling of skin tissue, and assists in healing bruised tissue; derived from the European arnica montana flowering plant with large yellow capitula

astaxanthin (BioAstin): enhances immune response and reduces inflammation; from the micro algae *H. pluvialis*, grown in Hawaii

azelaic acid: a pigment emulsifier (a skin-lightening agent); an exfoliant and pH adjustor; derived from oleic acid (unsaturated fatty acid) found in milk fats and potatoes

bellis perennis (daisy) flower extract (belidides): a very efficient natural skin-lightening agent that works by influencing various pathways involved in melanin production; derived from flowers of *bellis perennis* (the daisy flower)

bergamot: See *citrus aurantium bergamia fruit oil*

beta hydroxy acids (BHAs): a group of acids used in skin care preparations to assist in cellular turnover; salicylic acid is a BHA

beta glycans: See *cassia angustifolia seed polysaccharide*

BioAstin: See *astaxanthin*

biopein: a natural preservative made up of oregano leaf extract, thyme leaf extract, cinnamon bark extract, rosemary leaf extract, lavender leaf extract, and goldenseal root extract

borage: See *borago officinalis seed oil*

borago officinalis seed oil (borage): high in gamma linolenic and linoleic acid, borage oil is an essential fatty acid that increases ceramides in the skin by five times during one week's use; also boosts the skin's natural barrier functions; rich in vitamin C, calcium, and potassium

boswellia acids/boswellia serrata oil (frankincense): a group of compounds present in Indian frankincense extract that have potent anti-inflammatory properties, used to alleviate arthritis since biblical times

bromelain: keratin- (protein-) digesting enzyme from pineapple

butcher's broom: See *ruscus aculeatus root extract*

butyrospermum parkii (shea butter): a moisturizing, soothing emollient fat with cellular renewal properties; from the karite nut tree

calendula officinalis flower extract (marigold): an anti-inflammatory and antioxidant, commonly used to treat problem and acne skin; from the marigold flower

camu camu: See *myrciaria dubia*

cananga odorata oil (ylang ylang): promotes balancing of skin oils, relieves tension, reduces oil, softens, smoothes, rejuvenates, calms, and soothes; effective in the treatment of acne and eczema due to its ability to relieve stress common in these disorders

cannibis sativa l. seed oil (hemp oil): oil from hemp plants containing low levels of THC; a rich source of many of the fatty acids the skin uses; is suitable for dry skin applications

carnisine: a powerful antioxidant

carrageenan: See *chondrus crispus*

cassia angustifolia seed polysaccharide (beta glycans): retains moisture in the skin and leaves the skin like velvet; from seeds of the cassia augustifolia vahl fruit

centella asiatica extract (gotu kola) (hydrocotyl or Indian pennywort): called the "longevity plant" because of its ability to speed cellular renewal; from India

cereus grandiflorus (cactus) flower extract: has a unique ability to prevent moisture (water) loss from the stratum corneum, which regulates skin's water retention and evaporation; antioxidants in cactus flower extract also have cellular renewal properties

cholesteryl stearate/carbonate complex (liquid crystal): a protective and moisturizing emollient; from vegetable oil

chondrus crispus (carrageenan): a simple sugar, from seaweed, that detoxifies and tones the skin

citrus aurantium bergamia fruit oil (bergamot): has a sweet, fruity odor with an uplifting effect

citrus aurantium oil (neroli oil): suitable for the care of every skin type, including sensitive and inflamed skin, neroli oil supports the skin's renewal process of shedding old skin and stimulating new cell growth; from the orange blossom

citrus grandis extract (grapefruit extract): has antibacterial and antioxidant properties when used topically

citrus grandis peel oil (grapefruit): this oil has a light, fruity, fresh aroma that stimulates neurotransmitters and induces a slight euphoria; promotes renewed zest for life, lightness, and well-being

citrus limon oil (lemon) (organic): an antibacterial and antiseptic

citrus tangerine oil (tangerine): this sweet, sparkling fresh, lively aroma inspires, strengthens, and cheers one's spirits

cloudberry seed oil: See *rubus chamaemorus seed oil*

coenzyme Q-10 (CoQ$_{10}$ and ubiquinone): present in all living things, this powerful antioxidant prevents free radical damage

collinsonia canadensis (stone root): used externally, especially the leaves, for poultices and fomentations, bruises, wounds, sores, and cuts; the root contains resin, starch, mucilage, and wax; resin, tannin, wax, and volatile oil are found in the leaves; active chemicals in stone root include caryophyllene, delta cadinene, and elemicin, which provide antibacterial, antiedemic, anti-inflammatory, fungicidal, and antihistaminic properties

copper peptides: copper is a trace element found in every cell; in topical formulations, it is combined with small protein fragments, called peptides. Copper peptides enhance wound healing; promote collagen and elastin production to revive dull, lifeless skin; help erase fine lines and wrinkles; and restore moisture and firmness to the skin.

cranberry: See *vaccinium macrocarpon*

cucumis sativus oil (cucumber): with moisture-binding, tightening, and refreshing properties, this is good for relieving puffy eyes

cucurbita pepo enzymes (pumpkin): an exfoliant, with skin-softening properties

cucurbita pepo extract (pumpkin): a nutrient-dense pulp with enzymes containing a high concentration of vitamin A to promote skin renewal and healing

cucurbita pepo purée (pumpkin): a nutrient-dense pulp, containing a high concentration of vitamin A; a great source of retinol

cucurbita pepo seed oil (pumpkin): an excellent source of minerals (especially zinc) and essential fatty acids that help regulate sebum production; helps skin renew as it moisturizes

cucurbita pepo seed tar (pumpkin): a safer and more effective substitute for the commonly used coal tar; contains vitamin A derivatives, made more effective with its own botanically based hydrocarbons

cucurbita pepo wine (pumpkin): an antioxidant- and nutrient-rich wine from enzymatically predigested pumpkins

curcuma longa root extract (turmeric): a yellow coloring agent with anti-inflammatory and antioxidant properties; derived from an East Indian herb

cymbopogon schoenanthus oil (lemongrass): an essential oil from lemongrass that has purifying, refreshing, and hydrating effects

D_2O (heavy water): naturally occurring in saline lakes and in deep sea water, this bonds more strongly than regular water with the skin and other connective tissue, preventing the skin from drying out as quickly or as deeply; has remarkable protective and preserving action on tissue

D-alpha tocopherol (vitamin E): a powerful antioxidant and free radical scavenger, this is one of nature's most dynamic moisturizers. It aids cellular renewal, has healing properties, and improves skin elasticity, firmness, and tone. Vitamin E is a major antioxidant, which retards cellular aging due to oxidation. Made from vegetable sources, it repairs and prevents damage to the skin, and is excellent for healing cuts and scars.

D-beta fructan: this amino sugar escorts Vitamin C to the cells, promotes better-quality collagen and elastin, supplies nitrogen to the skin, strengthens the skin's immune cells, bolsters the skin's ability to moisturize, strengthen, and generally defend itself; derived from glucose molecules of the date palm

D-beta glucosamine: applied topically, D-beta glucosamine alleviates skin dryness, and facilitates exfoliation; due to its molecular weight, it penetrates deeply, making it very effective as a "building block" for collagen production; from Chinese foxglove, grain, and lichen

D-biotin: a B vitamin that promotes healing of acne

D-ceramides (sphingolipids): a skin conditioner that provides a protective skin barrier, repairing and hydrating

D-glucuronic acid: a precursor of vitamin C and a humectant

D-panthenol (pro-vitamin B_5): part of the water-soluble vitamin B complex (B_5); acts as a penetrating moisturizer

dunaliella sallina (algae extract): derived from the micro alga dunaliella salina, whose natural habitat is in salt lakes with a salinity nine times higher that other sources of saltwater

epidermal growth factor (EGF): a polypeptide (a protein molecule) that stimulates cell repair; derived from yeast

epigallocatechin gallate (EGCG from green tea): active constituents in green tea are the catechin polyphenols called epigallocatechin gallate (EGCG). Green tea catechins are potent antioxidants.

ethylhexyl palmitate, tribehenin, sorbitan isostearate, palmitoyl oligopeptide: a clinically tested peptide (chain of amino acids joined by a protein bond) that stimulates collagen and hyaluronic acid synthesis to achieve clearly defined, less wrinkled, and more voluptuous lips over the course of a 29-day treatment

euterpe oleracea (acai) fruit extract: this Amazonian fruit with powerful antioxidant properties is 20 times more powerful than the antioxidants found in red wine

frankincense: See *boswellia acids/boswellia serrata oil*

eyeseryl: has anti-edema properties; has been shown to be effective in reducing puffy eyes

fruit enzymes: with skin-refining properties, these protein- (keratin-) digesting enzymes have the ability to digest dead skin cells on the surface of the skin, revealing a smoother, fresher appearance

fucus vesiculosus algin (algae extract): inhibits the formation of the enzyme collagenase, which causes the degradation of collagen

gallic acid: abundantly present in the leaves of witch hazel, the flower of mango, the fruit of emblica or alma, pomegranate, gall oak, rhubarb, soybean, sumac tea leaves, and oak bark; gallic acid has antibacterial and antiviral properties and is a cancer preventative; also a skin lightener, which inhibits tyrosinase, decreasing melanin synthesis

garcinia indica (kokum): an emollient and stabilizer; derived from seeds of the garcinia indica tree in India

garcinia mangostana (mangosteen) peel powder: a powerful antioxidant and anti-inflammatory that relieves symptoms associated with eczema

ginkgo bilboa (ginkgo): a powerful antioxidant with detoxifying properties that revitalizes, stimulates and firms the skin; found to improve circulation by helping to increase healthy blood flow to the skin; known for its anti-aging properties; from the sacred chinese ginkgo tree

ginseng: See *panax ginseng*

glycolic acid: glycolic acid dissolves the binders (glue) that hold dead skin cells together; an AHA (alpha hydroxy acid) from rhubarb

glycyrrhiza glabra root extract (licorice): an anti-inflammatory, antioxidant, and skin lightener

gotu kola: See *centella asiatica extract*

grape seed extract: See *vitis vinifera seed extract*

grape seed oil: See *vitis vinifera oil*

hamamelis virginiana (witch hazel) water: has antihistaminic, antioxidant, anti-inflammatory, and antibacterial properties; derived from the hamamelis virginia, or witch hazel, tree

heavy water: See *D_2O*

hemp oil: See *cannibis sativa l. seed oil*

honeysuckle: See *lonicera caprifolium*

hydroxy propyl beta cyclodextrin (HPBCD): a botanical starch that improves firmness of the skin

jojoba: See *simmondsia chinensis beads*

kokum: See *garcinia indica*

L-arbutin: a naturally occurring form of hydroquinone; derived from bearberry extract (aka uva ursi)

L-arginine: an essential amino acid, which acts as a hydrator and antioxidant

L-ascorbic acid (vitamin C): a powerful antioxidant; the chirally correct form of vitamin C that assists in the production of collagen (must be formulated with at least 10% L-ascorbic acid to be effective)

L-glutathione: a glutamine-cysteine peptide, from purslane and spinach; left-handed for greater protection of membrane lipids from free radicals

L-lactic acid: naturally occurring in the human body, L-lactic acid is an alpha hydroxy acid (AHA) obtained from sour milk; because it has a larger molecule than glycolic acid, it may not be as irritating as other AHAs; enhances shedding of the outer layer of the skin and evenly thins the stratum corneum; gently clarifying for blemish-prone skin

L-limonene: an antibacterial that promotes oxygen penetration through the skin; an essential oil derived from star anis, buchu leaves, caraway, celery, and oranges

L-malic acid: an AHA that enhances shedding of the outer layer of the skin and improves the appearance of the skin; derived from apples and grapes

L-mandelic acid: a humectant, skin conditioner, and antioxidant; derived from bitter almond

L-proline: a left-handed amino acid that improves the strength of the cell envelope while keeping it elastic

L-sodium hyaluronate: hyaluronic acid in chiral form, this powerful humectant draws water from the ambient air and protects cells from rapid dehydration. This amino sugar is a component of hyaluronic acid, one of the glycosaminoglycans (polysaccharide chains) that make up the extracellular matrix (ground substance) of the dermis, which contains elastin and collagen. These compounds bind with water and help maintain the water and salt balance of the skin and keep the epidermis in tighter alignment with the dermis. Derived from Chinese Foxglove, grain, and lichen.

L-sodium PCA (sodium-2pyrrolidone carboxylate): has superhydrating effects for the skin, as it draws moisture from the air; derived from molasses

L-superoxide dismutase: this chirally correct antioxidant enzyme combines with the trace mineral selenium, found in the skin, and helps prevent oxidative damage to the skin; together they turn free radicals into harmless alcohol

L-tartaric acid: a powerful antioxidant from wine; enhances the effects of malic acid

lavendula angustifolia flower oil (lavender) (organic): an excellent source of zinc and essential fatty acids; helps skin renew as it moisturizes

lemongrass: See *cymbopogon schoenanthus oil*

licorice: See *glycyrrhiza glabra root extract*

limnanthes alba benth seed oil (meadowfoam): a small herbaceous winter-spring annual, originating in northern California and southern Oregon; highly emollient and soothing, penetrates quickly, with very high EFA levels

lonicera caprifolium (honeysuckle) flower extract: a natural antimicrobial, used to preserve skin care formulas

lycopene: a powerful antioxidant and anticarcinogenic; enhances communications between cells in the organs and tissues

macrocystis pyrifera extract (antarctic seaweed): with high iodine and sulfur amino acid content, this extract promotes anti-inflammatory and disinfectant actions, while moisturizing; its properties are attributed to its ability to react with protein and form a protective gel on the skin's surface; derived from seaweed prevalent in the Antarctic Sea

mallow extract: See *malva sylvestris extract*

malva sylvestris extract (mallow extract): an anti-inflammatory, soothing, refreshing emollient with high mucilage content; when in contact with water, it produces a soothing protective gel

mangosteen: See *garcinia mangostana*

meadowfoam: See *limnanthes alba benth seed oil*

melaleuca alternifolia essential oil (tea tree oil): an antibacterial and antifungal

morus alba (white mulberry) bark extract: a source of betulinic acid, which decreases ultraviolet-induced DNA breakage, resulting in melanoma; inhibits tumor development induced by carcinogenic chemicals; is an anti-inflammatory and antiviral, an inhibitor of prostaglandin synthesis, and an inhibitor of photoaging

myrciaria dubia (camu camu) fruit extract: high in flavonoids, this is the highest documented vitamin C–containing fruit on earth

myrtle: an anti-aging ingredient that delays cellular senescence (the process of growing old) and limits dermal degeneration (skin aging)

neroli oil: See *citrus aurantium oil*

niacinamide: vitamin B_3 in its more water-soluble form; topical application will decrease pruritus and inflammation, help acne-affected skin, decrease oiliness, alleviate atopic dermatitis, decrease UV-induced skin cancers, and help decrease facial pigmentation

olea europaea leaf extract (olive): a great carrier oil with excellent lubricating qualities and powerful antioxidants

palmitoyl tripeptide-5 (SYN-COLL): stimulates collagen synthesis, actively removes wrinkles, and has skin-firming and moisturizing properties

palmitoyl tripeptide diaminobutyloylhydroxythreonine, palmitoyl dipeptide diaminohydroxybutyrate (SYN-TACKS): this combination of two peptides stimulates proteins in the dermal-epidermal junction (DEJ); also improves structural integrity, epidermal nourishment, and molecular communication within the skin

panax ginseng (ginseng): an ancient whole body tonic, ginseng contains several organic compounds with antioxidant effects; when applied to the skin, it has been shown to enhance the cellular function of skin cells and stimulate skin cell regeneration; useful in combating wrinkles and the visible signs of aging

passiflora incarnata extract (passion flower): an antioxidant, with soothing properties

passion flower: See *passiflora incarnata extract*

patchouli: See *pogostemon cablin essential oil*

PBN (phenyl butyl nitrone or spin traps): a very powerful antioxidant; instead of destroying rogue oxygen molecules (free radicals), it traps them, then exports them into the respiratory cycle, where they are utilized in tissue respiration

pelargonium graveolens flower oil (geranium): a refreshing anti-irritant; derived from the geranium plant

phenethyl alcohol & caprylyl glycol (stabil preservative): together, these two substances constitute a compound called *stabil*, a globally approved and accepted nonsensitizing/nontoxic compound with broad-spectrum antimicrobial properties; it is so safe that it has been allowed to assert that it's "preservative free"

phospholipids: reduce moisture loss in the skin; carriers for deep penetration; derived from plants

pisum sativum (pea) extract (Proteasyl TP peptide): a protector of dermal proteins (collagen); this has anti-elastase, anticollagenase, and anti–free radical properties; protects and repairs epidermal proteins, and strengthens skins elasticity

pogostemon cablin essential oil (patchouli): balances oily/acne-prone skin

pomegranate: See *punica granatum extract*

porphyra umbilicalis extract (red algae): contains the same essential nutrients, trace elements, and amino acids present in human blood plasma; speeds the elimination of toxins from cells and acts as a natural cellular-renewal ingredient

Proteasyl TP peptide: See *pisum sativum (pea) extract*

pro-vitamin B$_5$: See *D-panthenol*

pseudoalteromas ferment extract (antarcticine): increases collagen and elastin production while protecting the skin from extreme cold, and preventing dryness of the skin; derived from the Antarctic Sea

pumpkin: See *cucurbita*

punica granatum extract (pomegranate): a powerful antioxidant

pyrus malus fruit extract (apple) (Applephenon™): a fantastic skin-lightening ingredient; inhibits production of tyrosine and melanin

R-lipoic acid: a powerful water- and oil-soluble antioxidant, 400 times more powerful than vitamin C as an antioxidant; increases glutathione, the body's most important antioxidant; a powerful anti-inflammatory as well

red algae: See *porphyra umbilicalis extract*

resveratrol: a phytoalexin, which is an antibiotic produced by a plant's defense system in response to environmental, insect, or animal stress; works as an antioxidant, an anti-inflammatory, and an vasodilator; stimulates cellular proliferation and collagen synthesis; and blocks the deleterious effects from UVB radiation; derived from red grape skins, pine nuts, and the root of polygonum cuspidatum

rosa affinis rubiginosa seed oil (rose hips): particularly rich in essential fatty acids (EFAs), known to be necessary constituents of cell membranes in the synthesis of hormones like prostaglandins for skin welfare

rose hips: See *rosa affinis rubiginosa seed oil*

rubus chamaemorus seed oil (cloudberry seed oil): consists of essential linoleic and alpha linoleic acids, UV-protecting carotenoids, and membrane-strengthening phytosterols; contains free vitamin E, easily absorbed by the skin

rubus idaeus rosaceae fruit extract (raspberry extract): an antiseptic and antibacterial

ruscus aculeatus root extract (butcher's broom): increases circulation and inhibits inflammation; derived from a shrub native to Europe

salicylic acid: softens the skin's barrier cells; an antibacterial that helps eliminate clogged pores; a beta hydroxy acid responsible for oxygenating and detoxifying; derived from pumpkin seeds

salix alba bark extract (white willow): an anti-inflammatory and a pain reliever

sandalwood: See *santalum album oil*

santalum album oil (sandalwood): an essential oil that has calming, harmonizing, and balancing effects; acts in deep, slow waves, embracing emotions with a warm, woody fragrance

shea butter: See *butyrospermum parkii*

simmondsia chinensis beads (jojoba): exfoliating beads that loosen and lift away dead skin cells without damaging skin; derived from the jojoba plant

simmondsia chinensis oil (jojoba): a thick waxy oil from jojoba beans that promotes cellular renewal and is a great moisturizer; effectively penetrates human skin due to its similarity to human sebum

sodium-2pyrrolidone carboxylate: See *L-sodium PCA*

sphingolipids: See *D-ceramides*

spin traps: See *PBN (phenyl butyl nitrone)*

squalane: a lipid similar to what the body produces naturally to lubricate and heal; has moisturizing and lubricating properties; may reduce skin irritation and allergic responses; derived from Spanish olives

stabil preservative: See *phenethyl alcohol* & *caprylyl glycol*

stone root: See *collinsonia canadensis*

symphytum officinale (allantoin): healing, soothing, and believed to aid in the healing of damaged skin by stimulating new tissue growth; derived from the comfrey root

SYN-COLL: See *palmitoyl tripeptide-5*

SYN-TACKS: See *palmitoyl tripeptide diaminobutyloylhydroxythreonine, palmitoyl dipeptide diaminohydroxybutyrate*

tea tree oil: See *melaleuca alternifolia essential oil*

thermus thermophilus ferment (Venuceane): a powerful antioxidant, activated by heat and light, that protects against UV damage, stimulates skin cell differentiation and maturation, and strengthens the stratum corneum to make it more resistant to assault

titanium dioxide (TiO2): a naturally occurring compound, which is mined; the "natural" choice for a physical sunblock because it is more cosmetically pleasing than zinc oxide; performs as both a UVA and a UVB protectant (protects against skin cancer and wrinkling due to sun exposure); also used for cosmetic reasons; imparts a sheen to the lips and gives body and texture to products

tocotrienols (D-gamma, D-alpha): powerful antioxidants

totarol: an extract of the New Zealand totara tree with potent antibacterial and antioxidant properties; propionium bacterium, the bacterium involved in acne, is particularly sensitive to this extract; effective in the treatment of acne and rosacea

turmeric: See *curcuma longa root extract*

ubiquinone: See *coenzyme Q-10*

vaccinium corymbosum l. ericaceae extract (blueberry) purée (or pulp): soothing, with a high concentration of antioxidants

vaccinium macrocarpon (cranberry): an antibacterial and an antioxidant that nourishes skin; derived from cranberries

Venuceane: See *thermus thermophilus ferment*

vitamin C: See *L-ascorbic acid*

vitamin E: See *D-alpha tocopherol*

vitis vinifera oil (grape seed oil): a powerful antioxidant that quickly penetrates the skin; rich in flavonoids; inhibits allergic reactions; protects skin's own collagen, elastin, and hyaluronic acid

vitis vinifera seed extract (grape seed extract): a counterirritant with soothing antibacterial properties

vitus vinifera seed extract (red grape extract): a potent antioxidant; strong polyphenol content

white mulberry: See *morus alba*

white willow: See *salix alba bark extract*

witch hazel: See *hamamelis virginiana*

ylang ylang: See *cananga odorata oil*

yucca schidigera leaf extract (yucca, Mojave yucca, Spanish dagger, and yucca aloifolia): has gentle, nontoxic foaming properties as well as emollient effects; Native Americans used yucca to make soap

zea mays silk extract (corn): a natural emollient, derived from fine corn silk

ZinClear: a physical (reflective) sunblock that blocks UVA and UVB radiation

zingiver officinale root extract (ginger): an anti-inflammatory and warming substance that increases circulation

APPENDIX C

Toxic Ingredients

acetone: Acetone is an irritant and inhalation may lead to hepatotoxic effects (causing liver damage). The vapors should be avoided, and under no circumstances should it be consumed directly or indirectly. The most familiar household use of acetone is as the active ingredient in nail polish remover. Acetone is also used to make plastic, fibers, drugs, and other chemicals.

aldehydes: See *formaldahyde.*

aluminum: Has been linked to Alzheimer's disease.

artificial (synthetic) colors: Labeled FD&C (Food, Drug or Cosmetics) or D&C (Drugs or Cosmetics), this designation is followed by a color and then a number (FD&C Red No. 6, D&C Green No. 6, or FD&C Blue No. 1). Artificial colors are made from coal tar, a derivative of coal. There is a great deal of controversy about the use of coal tars. Almost all the coal tar colors cause cancer. Some artificial colors even contain heavy-metal impurities, such as arsenic and lead, which are known carcinogens.

benzalkonium chloride: A preservative that can cause allergic reactions.

benzene: A carcinogen whose use as an additive in gasoline is now limited, but it is an important industrial solvent and precursor in the production of drugs, plastics, synthetic rubber, and dyes. Benzene is a natural constituent of crude oil, but it is usually synthesized from other compounds present in petroleum.

benzoyl peroxide: Jack Breitbart of Revlon laboratories first developed benzoyl peroxide for use in treating acne in the 1920s. It is typically placed over the affected areas in gel or cream form, in concentrations of 2.5% increasing through the usually effective 5% to up to 10%. Pure benzoyl peroxide is highly flammable, explosive, toxic and a possible tumor promoter and may act as a mutagen, and should be handled with care. Benzoyl peroxide removes the top layer of skin, which caused photosensitivity; sun protection (sunblocks, sunscreen, or clothing that blocks the sun's rays) must be worn to protect vulnerable, unprotected skin. Sunburn and premature aging is a risk if sun protection is not worn.

coal tar: A brown or black liquid of high viscosity, which smells of naphthalene and aromatic hydrocarbons, coal tar is among the by-products when coal is carbonized to make coke or gasified to make coal gas. Coal tars are complex and variable mixtures of phenols, polycyclic aromatic hydrocarbons (PAHs), and heterocyclic compounds.

diethanolamine (DEA), triethanolamine (TEA), monoethanolamine (MEA): Used in cosmetics as emulsifiers and/or foaming agents. DEA, TEA, and MEA are "amines" (ammonia compounds) and can produce cancer-causing nitrosamines when they come into contact with nitrates.

ethylenediamine: This corrosive and toxic substance causes severe irritation with redness, pain, and possibly burns, according to the Material Data Safety Sheet (MSDS). Ethylenediamine may be absorbed through the skin, and it may cause allergic reaction in sensitive individuals.

ethylenediaminetetraacetic acid (EDTA): EDTA is used as a preservative in food and it's commonly found in cosmetic formulations. In cosmetics, it acts as a preservative and chelating agent (a chemical that combines with a metal to form a new chemical compound). Drug warning: Direct contact with EDTA may cause dermal sensitization (eczema) or allergic conjunctivitis.

formaldehyde: Formaldehyde is a known cancer-causing agent (carcinogen). It also causes allergic reactions, sometimes aggravating and provoking contact dermatitis, headaches, and chronic fatigue. The vapor, if inhaled, is extremely irritating to the eyes, nose, and throat.

fragrances (synthetic): The most common cause of allergies and irritant reactions to cosmetics, synthetic fragrances are estrogen disrupters. The FDA does not require manufacturers to list the ingredients of a "fragrance." Fragrances may contain as many as 4,000 separate chemicals.

isopropyl alcohol: Derived from petroleum, this is used in antifreeze, shellac, and body care products. Side effects include headache, dizziness, depression, nausea, vomiting, and coma. It penetrates the skin easily and can destroy intestinal flora, leaving the body's major organs open to parasites, as well as triggering cancers.

Isopropyl alcohol isn't needed in body care formulations, but the petroleum industry makes a ton of money off this industrial by-product.

isotretinoin: Isotretinoin, a medication used for the treatment of severe acne, is sometimes used in the prevention and treatment of certain skin cancers. It is a retinoid, meaning it is derived from vitamin A and is found in small quantities naturally in the body. Oral isotretinoin is marketed under many different trade names, most commonly Accutane (Roche), Amnesteem (Mylan), Claravis (Barr), Decutan (Actavis), Isotane (Pacific Pharmaceuticals), Sotret (Ranbaxy), Oratane (Genepharm Australasia) or Roaccutane (Roche). Topical isotretinoin is most commonly marketed under the trade names Isotrex or Isotrexin (Stiefel). Ad-verse drug reactions associated with isotretinoin therapy include the following:

- Common: mild acne flare-up; dryness of skin, lips, and mucous membranes; infection of the cuticles; cheilitis; itching; skin fragility; skin peeling; rashes; flushing; photosensitivity; nosebleeds; dry eyes, eye irritation, conjunctivitis, and reduced tolerance to contact lenses; raised liver enzymes; headaches; hair thinning; myalgia, and/or arthralgia.

- Infrequent: severe acne flare-up, raised blood glucose level, overall inflammation in the body, fatigue.

- Rare: impaired night vision, cataracts, optic neuritis, menstrual disturbances, inflammatory bowel disease, pancreatitis, hepatitis, corneal opacities, papilloedema, idiopathic intracranial hypertension, and skeletal hyperostosis. It is also believed that isotretinoin therapy may cause severe depression, although there is no conclusive evidence for this.

lanolin: Made from the fatty secretions of sheep's wool, lanolin cannot be used in its pure from because of its allergy-causing potential. Cosmetic-grade lanolin may be contaminated with carcinogenic pesticides, such as dieldrin, lindane, and DDT.

mineral oil: A liquid mixture of hydrocarbons obtained from petroleum, mineral oil can attract dirt and causes clogged pores. Derived from petroleum, which is the chief reason for the greasy after-feel on the skin, it slows the skin's natural cell development, causing the skin to age prematurely.

MEA (monoethanolamine): Used in skin care formulas to adjust pH.

nitrosamines: Produced from nitrites and secondary amines, which often occur in the form of proteins, nitrosamines can cause cancers in a wide variety of animal species; this suggests that they may also be carcinogenic in humans.

octyl dimethyl PABA (padimate-O and p-aminobenzoic acid): PABA is used in sunscreens, and can cause skin irritations.

PABA: See *octyl dimethyl PABA*

parabens (methyl-, propyl-, butyl-, and ethyl-): A universally used preservative with estrogenic properties.

persistent organic pollutants (POPs): These chemical substances persist in the environment, bioaccumulate through the food web, and pose a risk of causing adverse effects to human health and the environment.

petrolatum (petroleum jelly): A grease made from petroleum, this is used in industry because it is unbelievably cheap. Petrolatum exhibits many of the same potentially harmful properties as mineral oil. While attempting to hold moisture in your skin, it traps the toxins and wastes that are inside your skin's layers. This occlusive substance suffocates your skin, interfering with tissue respiration, which leads to prematurely aged skin.

phenylenediamine (PPD): PPD is a chemical substance that is universally used as a permanent hair dye. It may also be found in textile or fur dyes, dark-colored cosmetics, temporary tattoos, photographic developer and lithography plates, photocopying and printing inks, black rubber, oils, greases, and gasoline. The most common mild reaction to hair dye with PPD is dermatitis to the upper eyelids or the rims of the ears. In more severe cases, there may be marked reddening and swelling of the scalp and the face. The eyelids may completely close and the allergic contact dermatitis reaction may become widespread. Professionals working with PPD, such as hairdressers and film developers, may develop dermatitis on their hands.

phthalates: Phthalates, or phthalate esters, are a group of chemical compounds that are predominantly used as plasticizers (substances added to plastics to increase their flexibility). They are mostly used to turn polyvinyl chloride from a hard plastic into a softer, flexible plastic. Phthalates are also used in nail polish, hair spray, and perfumes, and have estrogen-disrupting properties. Phthalates have been shown to build up in fatty tissue and negatively influence endocrine function.

polyethylene glycol (PEG): This carcinogenic ingredient, derived from petroleum, can reduce the skin's moisture retention. It's used in caustic oven cleansers to cut grease and in cosmetic formulations to adjust the viscosity.

propylene glycol (PG): Commonly used in moisturizers as a humectant, PG is the main active ingredient in antifreeze, and may also be found in brake and hydraulic fluids. It is also used in food processing. The EPA requires workers in direct contact with PG to wear protective gloves, clothing, and goggles. Direct contact can cause brain, liver, and kidney abnormalities. Many stick deodorants have higher concentrations of PG than is allowed for most industrial use. The Material Data Safety Sheet (MSDS) warns formulators who use propylene glycol about the following potential hazards:

• May cause skin and eye irritation.

• May be harmful if inhaled or ingested.

• Can cause nausea, vomiting, headaches, gastrointestinal disturbances, and depression.

• Can inhibit skin cell growth. This means that your cells will not be able to reproduce normally. If your body cannot make new cells, then the cells will get old and wrinkled. Did you know that some wrinkle creams can make you look older, rather than younger? Propylene glycol in their formulation may account for that.

• Can damage the skin and muscle tissue. The Environmental Protection Agency (EPA) requires food workers to wear protective gloves, clothing, and goggles when working with PG because this substance is absorbed into the skin very quickly.

• Is linked to contact dermatitis, liver and brain abnormalities, and kidney damage.

quaternium 15: Used as a preservative in cosmetics and toiletry items, as well as skin moisturizers and hair care products, this compound commonly causes allergic reactions and dermatitis, and breaks down into formaldehyde.

sodium cyanide: This is a highly toxic chemical compound, also known as *sodium salt of hydrocyanic acid* and *cyanogran*. Cyanide salts are among the most rapidly acting of all known poisons. Cyanide is a potent inhibitor of respiration. Initially, acute cyanide poisoning results in a red or ruddy complexion in the victim because the tissues are not able to use the oxygen in the blood.

sodium lauryl (laureth) sulfate: This widely used detergent (foaming agent) is used in industrial engine degreasers, garage-floor cleaners, water softeners, and auto-cleaning products, as well as many skin and hair care products. It is often disguised in so-called "natural" products as (in parentheses) as a coconut derivative. According to the *Journal of the American College of Toxicology*, sodium lauryl sulfate corrodes and damages the hair follicles and can actually cause your hair to fall out! Sodium lauryl sulfate can stay in your body for up to seven days. According to the American Academy of Dermatology (www.aad.org), these surfactant molecules stay on your skin long after you think you've washed them off and as they sit there, they literally strip fatty acids, moisture, and amino acids from your hair and skin.

stearalkonium chloride: Used in hair conditioners and creams, this chemical was first developed for the fabric industry as a fabric softener.

talc/talcum powder: Inhaling talc may cause acute respiratory distress and result in death. It also causes cancer in laboratory animals.

triclosan: Comonly used in antibacterial cleansers, toothpaste, and household products, triclosan is a synthetic antibacterial ingredient with a chemical structure similar to that of Agent Orange. The Environmental Protection Agency registers it as a pesticide, highly toxic to any living organism. It is also classified as a chlorophenol, a chemical class suspected of causing cancer in humans. Due to its hormone-disrupting potential, it may affect fertility and cause birth defects. Its manufacturing process produces dioxin, a powerful hormone-disrupting chemical with toxic effects in quantities as small as parts per trillion (that's one drop in 300 Olympic-size swimming pools). Triclosan is stored in body fat and can potentially accumulate to toxic levels in the kidneys, liver, and lungs. It may cause paralysis, suppression of the immune system, brain hemorrhages, and heart problems.

ureas (imidazolidinyl urea, diazolidinyl urea, and/or DMDM HydantoinP): The most commonly used cosmetic preservatives, after the parabens. They are just three of the many preservatives that release formaldehyde. According to the Mayo Clinic, formaldehyde can irritate the respiratory system, cause skin irritations, and trigger heart palpitations. Exposure to formaldehyde-releasing products may also cause allergies, congestion, nausea, headaches, dizziness, ear infections, chronic fatigue, depression, asthma, chest pains, and loss of sleep. But, more seriously, formaldehyde is toxic to the immune system, it mutates human cells, and it's carcinogenic.

Index

About the Authors

Myra Michelle Eby is a skin care expert with over 25 years' experience in the holistic wellness industry. She is the founder and president of MyChelle Dermaceuticals LLC (mychelleusa.com), a cruelty-free, eco-friendly skin care company that combines nature and science to create all-natural, nontoxic products. Committed to living green and giving back to the community, Myra sponsors the HopeFoal Project based in Boulder, Colorado, and donates a portion of her company's profits to the local animal shelter, Farm Sanctuary, and the Campaign to Label Genetically Engineered Foods. She has written numerous articles about natural, nontoxic skin care for national publications.

Karolyn A. Gazella, a cancer survivor, is the coauthor of the *Definitive Guide to Cancer: An Integrative Approach to Prevention, Treatment, and Healing*. She is the founding publisher of the journal *Integrative Medicine* and has written several books and hundreds of articles on the topic of natural health. She is also the executive director of the nonprofit organization Medicine Horse Program (www.medicinehorse.org), located in Boulder, Colorado, which is an innovative equine-assisted therapy program that helps high-risk youth.

www.ingramcontent.com/pod-product-compliance
Lightning Source LLC
Chambersburg PA
CBHW050222270326
41914CB00003BA/525

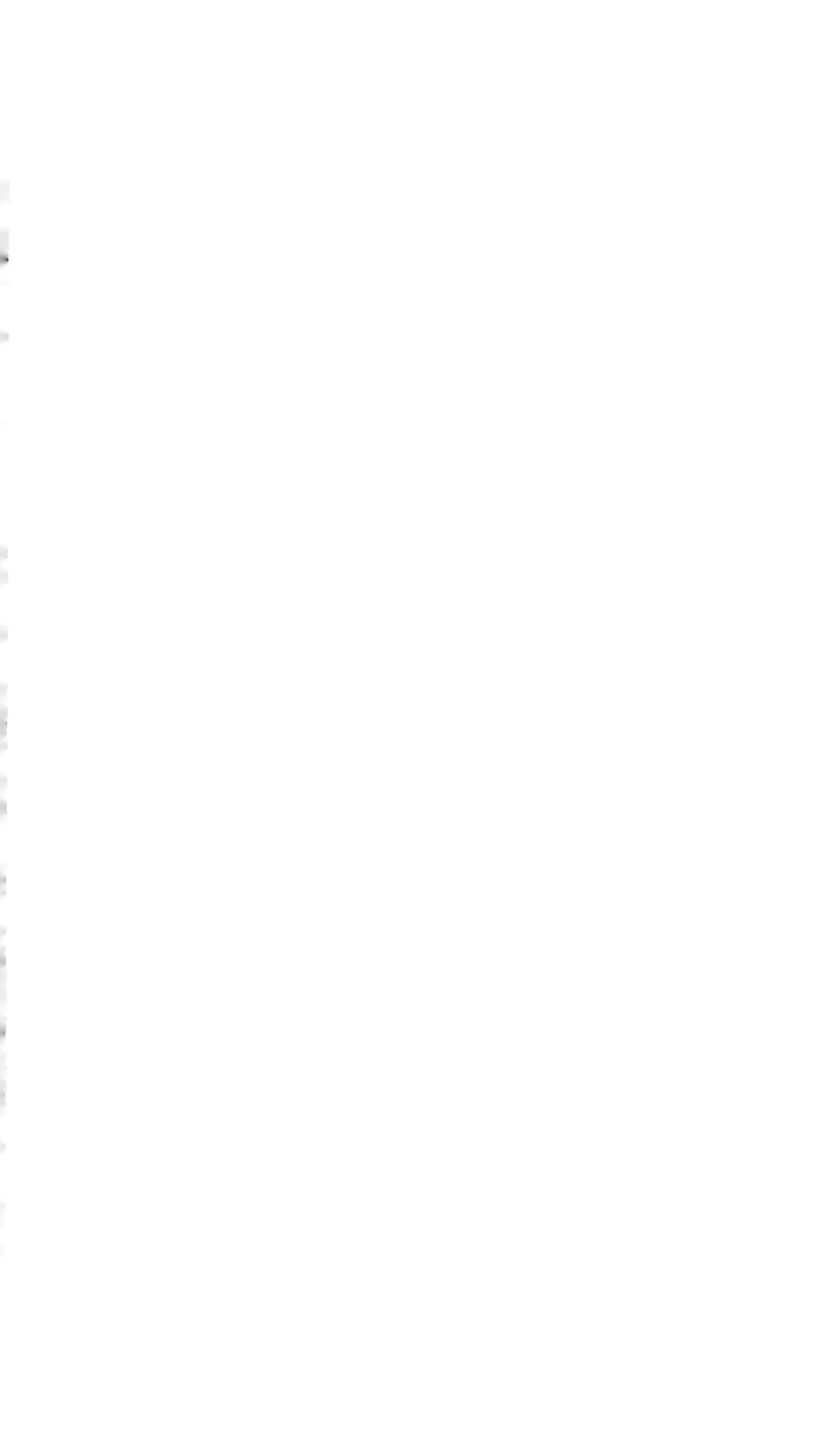